W. B. SAUNDERS COMPANY

Philadelphia • London • Toronto •
Mexico City • Rio de Janeiro •
Sydney • Tokyo • Hong Kong

1985

Paton and Goldberg's   SECOND EDITION

MANAGEMENT OF OCULAR INJURIES

THOMAS A. DEUTSCH, M.D.

Assistant Professor of Ophthalmology,
Rush Medical College; Assistant
Attending, Rush-Presbyterian-St. Luke's
Medical Center, Chicago, Illinois;
Formerly, Chief Resident in
Ophthalmology, University of Illinois
Eye and Ear Infirmary, Chicago, Illinois

DANIEL B. FELLER, M.D.

Attending Ophthalmologist, Prentice
Eye Institute, St Luke's Hospital
Medical Center, Phoenix, Arizona;
Formerly, Chief Resident in
Ophthalmology, University of Illinois
Eye and Ear Infirmary, Chicago, Illinois

W. B. Saunders Company: West Washington Square
Philadelphia, PA 19105

Library of Congress Cataloging in Publication Data

Paton, David.
Paton and Goldberg's Management of ocular injuries.

Bibliography: p.
Includes index.

1. Eye—Wounds and injuries.   I. Goldberg, Morton F.,
1937–   .   II. Deutsch, Thomas A.   III. Feller, Daniel
B.   IV. Title.   V. Title: Management of ocular injuries.
[DNLM: 1. Eye Injuries—diagnosis. 2. Eye Injuries—
therapy. WW 525 P312m]

RE831.P3 1985   617.7'13   85–2310
ISBN 0–7216–1173–7

Listed here is the latest translated edition of this book together with the language of the translation and the publisher.

Spanish (*1st Edition*)–Editorial JIMS, Barcelona, Spain

Paton & Goldberg's Management of Ocular Injuries   ISBN   0–7216–1173–7

Last digit is the print number: 9   8   7   6   5   4   3   2   1

To
Elise
and
Sharon

Foreword

Trauma to the eye is a perennial problem of major proportions. In 1968, the preface to the first version of this manual emphasized that "Modernization of society has clearly not lessened . . . accidental and intentional assaults on the human body; in many respects it has increased them." The passage of time has validated this assertion, underscoring the potential usefulness of this newest edition for emergency room physicians and nurses, as well as for practicing ophthalmologists.

The passage of time also has witnessed the emergence of "Hi-Tech" ophthalmic surgery, much of which is now routinely applied in the therapy of ocular trauma. Microsurgical techniques have become standardized and have spawned better suture material and needles, finer manual instruments, and a large variety of automated machines for intraocular use. These devices permit complex and precise techniques not possible when earlier versions of this book were written, but their availability has not eliminated the need for the triage health officer or the ophthalmic surgeon to think in terms of traditional and thoroughly tested surgical principles related to the eye. Thomas Deutsch and Daniel Feller have emphasized these timeless principles along with today's sophisticated technologic maneuvers. Their contributions have been essential in updating this basic book and have re-emphasized our initial and simple goal for it; namely, "the presentation of guidelines for clinical management of ocular trauma."

MORTON F. GOLDBERG, M.D.

Preface

This second edition, now titled *Paton and Goldberg's Management of Ocular Injuries*, was begun when we were still in training and on the faculty at the University of Illinois Eye and Ear Infirmary. We have both left that institution, but the principles first studied in the first edition of this manual continue to serve us.

Some aspects of ocular trauma management have changed dramatically in the nine years since the first edition was published, while others have remained the same. Vitrectomy, a new and promising technique in 1976, has now become a routine and indispensable tool. Antifibrinolytic agents have reduced the rate of secondary hemorrhage after traumatic hyphema to less than 10 per cent. The proliferation of CT scanners into even the smallest community hospitals has taken much of the guesswork out of trauma diagnosis. Despite these advances in the diagnosis and management of ocular injuries, the basic principle of carefully and completely closing the eye remains the primary goal in every penetrating injury.

The increasing usefulness of vitreous surgical techniques has spawned a cadre of ocular trauma specialists. That this group of surgeons is growing is testimony to the fact that ocular trauma continues to plague our communities. Indeed, while our reparative skills are ever increasing, our preventive skills continue to lag behind. All ophthalmologists must be prepared to handle at least some aspects of the care of these patients. It is for this reason that we have prepared a second edition of this manual.

THOMAS A. DEUTSCH, M.D.

DANIEL B. FELLER, M.D.

Contents

Preliminary Considerations

1.1 EVALUATION OF OCULAR INJURIES

Chemical burns of the eye and occlusion (or impending occlusion) of the central retinal artery are the two ocular emergencies that require *immediate* therapy. Endophthalmitis is next in priority for urgent management. Other conditions of primary concern are lacerations of the globe, intraocular foreign bodies, severe lid lacerations, orbital cellulitis, and hyphemas. Although this latter group of injuries requires prompt attention, therapy can be instituted within hours rather than minutes (Table 1–1); thus, there is usually time for adequate examination, unhurried decisions, and optimal preparation of treatment facilities.

Too often, lacerations of the globe are undetected because tightly swollen lids are not separated by lid retractors to yield an adequate view of the eye itself. Surgical correction of facial fractures is sometimes completed without recognition of a blow-out fracture of the orbital floor that was not visualized on routine skull films. Intraocular bleeding is occasionally unidentified, and persons with "black eyes" are simply dispatched with instructions for cold compresses. Minor lid lacerations are at times repaired without recognition of an intraocular foreign body

Table 1–1. OCULAR EMERGENCIES AND MEASURES TO AVOID

True emergencies. Therapy should be instituted within *minutes.*
1. Chemical burns of the cornea.
2. Central retinal artery occlusion.

Urgent situations. Therapy should be instituted within one to several *hours.*
1. Endophthalmitis.
2. Penetrating injuries of the globe.
3. Acute narrow-angle glaucoma (angle closure).
4. Pupillary-block glaucoma (lens or vitreous incarcerated in pupil); lens in anterior chamber.
5. Orbital cellulitis.
6. Cavernous sinus thrombosis.
7. Corneal ulcer.
8. Gonococcal conjunctivitis.
9. Corneal foreign body.
10. Corneal abrasion.
11. Acute iritis and formation of synechias.
12. Giant cell arteritis with acute ischemia of optic nerve.
13. *Acute* retinal tear with hemorrhage.
14. *Acute* retinal detachment.
15. *Acute* vitreous hemorrhage.
16. Descemetocele.
17. Hyphema.
18. Lid laceration.

Semi-urgent situations. Therapy should be instituted within *days* whenever possible or sometimes within weeks.
1. Optic neuritis.
2. Ocular tumors.
3. Exophthalmos, acute.
4. Previously undiagnosed chronic simple glaucoma.
5. Old retinal detachment.
6. Strabismic or other remediable amblyopias in very young children.
7. Blow-out fracture of the orbit.

Measures to avoid.
1. Anesthetic ointments. (Have too prolonged an effect; the patient may inadvertently traumatize himself.)
2. Any anesthetic given to a patient for output use. (The patient may become "addicted" or may injure himself inadvertently.)
3. Ointments of any kind:
    When penetrating trauma is present. (The ointment may get into the anterior chamber.)
    When fundus examination will be required. (The view of the fundus is mechanically obscured by the ointment.)
4. Atropine for routine use. (Shorter-acting cycloplegics such as tropicamide or cyclopentolate are frequently more desirable.)
5. Corticosteroids in any form:
    If diagnosis in uncertain.
    If fungal overgrowth or herpes simplex infection is likely.

or an ocular perforation. Compulsive examination of every patient with an ocular injury is necessary to avoid these oversights.

1.2 BASIC WORK-UP OF OCULAR INJURIES

A comprehensive examination of various types of injuries of the eye and its adnexal structures should include the items summarized in Table 1–2. Figure 1–1 shows the minimum equipment essential for emergency room evaluation of ocular trauma, and Figures 1–2 and 1–3 show minimal sets for minor surgical repairs.

Reduction of vision after an injury should be thoroughly evaluated according to the criteria listed in Table 1–3. The position of the eyes, lids,

Table 1–2. EMERGENCY ROOM EVALUATION OF TRAUMA AFFECTING LIDS, EYE, OR ORBIT

1. Obtain history of previous eye disorders, type of chemical burn or nature of injuring object, and history of tetanus immunization. Gas-gangrene panophthalmitis can still occur.*
2. Render first aid in case of true emergency (see Table 1–1).
3. Determine visual acuity and screen visual fields by confrontation with test object. Was patient wearing glasses when injured? Inspect glasses.
4. Differentiate partially and completely penetrating (perforating) injuries of cornea and sclera. Use lid retractors. Anesthetize orbicularis muscle if squeezing prevents atraumatic examination of eyeball. Note uveal, vitreal, or lenticular prolapse.
5. Note hemorrhages and infections of orbit, lids, or conjunctiva. Account for chemosis.
6. Investigate depth of all lid lacerations, noting fat in wound. Seek foreign bodies under lid: evert lid and sweep fornix with cotton swab after use of topical anesthetic.
7. Palpate orbital rim; feel for crepitus through lids; test facial and corneal sensation; auscultate for orbitocranial bruit.
8. Appraise real or apparent displacement of globe: anterior, posterior, or vertical. Use exophthalmometer.
9. Characterize diplopia by analysis of ocular ductions and versions; attempt forced-duction test using forceps and topical anesthetic.
10. Record pupil shape, size, and reactions. Is the Marcus Gunn phenomenon present?
11. Inspect for hyphema, iridodonesis, and iridodialysis.
12. Examine cornea for opacities, ulcers, foreign bodies, rust rings, and abrasions (use fluorescein paper); avoid medications containing steroids.
13. Use loupe or slit lamp to detect foreign-body paths in cornea, iris, or lens.
14. Estimate comparative depths of anterior chambers for evaluation of intumescent cataract, displaced lens, and a possibility of recessed chamber angle.
15. If traumatized globe is intact and cornea is undamaged, measure intraocular pressure with tonometer.
16. In ophthalmoscopic examination, differentiate various types of intraocular hemorrhage. Record appearance of nervehead, macula, and retinal circulation. Visualize foreign bodies if possible. Search for retinal tears and disinsertions before vitreous blood obscures them. Use indirect ophthalmoscope.
17. Obtain x-rays in all cases of possible retained foreign body in globe or orbit and whenever orbital fracture is conceivable.
18. Remember to culture all foreign bodies in contact with eye tissue (instead of taping to patient's chart).
19. Consider value of photographing all injuries.

*Bhargava SK, Chopdar A: Gas gangrene panophthalmitis. Br J Ophthalmol 55:136–138, 1971.

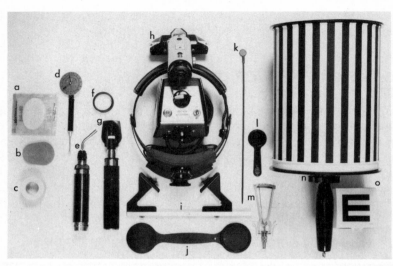

Figure 1–1. Basic equipment for examination of and first aid for ocular trauma: (a) sterile patch, (b) Elastoplast patch, (c) roll of Micropore paper tape, (d) ophthalmodynamometer, (e) transilluminator, (f) lens for indirect ophthalmoscope, (g) direct ophthalmoscope, (h) indirect ophthalmoscope, (i) exophthalmometer, (j) occluder and Maddox rod, (k) test object for confrontation fields, (l) multi-pinhole, (m) Schiötz tonometer, (n) drum to test optokinetic response, (o) E-game test box.

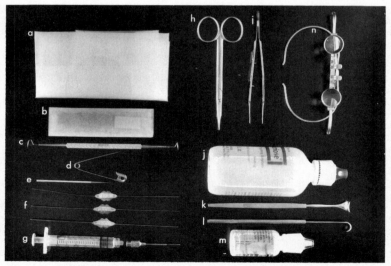

Figure 1–2. Basic equipment (continued): (a) plastic eye drape, (b) sterile fluorescein-impregnated paper strip, (c) Worst pigtail probe, (d) large safety pin for punctum dilatation, (e) punctum dilator, (f) Bowman probes, (g) small syringe and blunt-tipped needle, (h) utility scissors, (i) Castroviejo forceps (0.5 mm), (j) sterile irrigation solution in squeeze bottle, (k and l) Desmarres retractors, (m) topical anesthetic, (n) loupe.

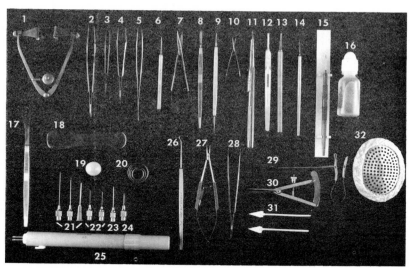

Figure 1–3. Basic equipment (continued): (1) Maumenee lid speculum, (2) Castroviejo forceps (0.12 mm), (3) Bonn forceps (0.12 mm), (4) McPherson tying forceps, (5) jeweler's forceps, (6) Barraquer iris sweep, (7) sharp-tipped Westcott scissors, (8) Tooke knife, (9) Martinez dissecting spatula, (10) Vannas scissors, (11) razor blade breaker-holder, (12) Bard-Parker blade holder, (13) Beaver blade and holder, (14) Franceschetti hook, (15) Ziegler knife, (16) sterile balanced salt solution, (17) orbital retractor, (18) lid plate for globe protection, (19) plastic shell to protect cornea, (20) Flieringa rings, (21) Atkinson needle, cystitome needle, and blunt No. 18 needle, (22) No. 27 and No. 30 irrigation cannulas, (23) Randolph cyclodialysis spatula, (24) short, blunt needle for lens aspiration, (25) disposable cautery, (26) muscle hook, (27) microsurgical needle holder, (28) Arruga lens forceps, (29) foreign body forceps, (30) measuring device, (31) Weck cellulose sponges, (32) Fox metal shield.

Table 1–3. PARTIAL DIFFERENTIAL DIAGNOSIS OF POST-TRAUMATIC LOSS OF VISION

1. Lid swelling; blood or foreign material covering cornea; corneal damage.
2. Hyphema; vitreous hemorrhage.
3. Traumatic cataract; luxation of lens.
4. Central retinal artery or vein occlusion (from markedly increased orbital pressure or embolus).
5. Traumatic retinal edema and hemorrhages of retina from direct or contrecoup blows.
6. Retinal detachment.
7. Avulsion of optic nerve by trauma of lateral orbital wall or contrecoup blow to head.
8. Indirect trauma to optic nerves and/or chiasm (traumatic optic neuritis).
9. Intracranial interruption of visual pathways (hemorrhage, foreign body).
10. Cortical blindness from hematoma, ischemia, or anoxia (patient may be unaware of blindness).
11. Acute congestive (angle-closure) glaucoma precipitated by emotional trauma of recent accident or from intumescent lens, etc.
12. Hysteria.
13. Malingering.

and pupils; the sensitivity of the corneas; and the presence of nystagmus, papilledema, or diplopia may help in evaluating possible neurologic disorders.

a. Evaluation of Visual Acuity

A knowledge of the patient's visual acuity is essential in planning a proper workup and management strategy. The best corrected distance visual acuity (or the acuity measured with a pinhole) should be determined in most cases. Occasionally, because of the patient's systemic condition, an approximation of the acuity may be obtained using a near acuity card. If the patient is unable to see the distance chart, the ability to count fingers at a distance (e.g., CF at 2 ft), to see hand motions (e.g., HM at 3 ft), or to perceive light is recorded. If the acuity is HM or worse, then the ability to project light in four quadrants is noted.

One must be especially clever when testing a child's acuity, as he or she often paradoxically tries to please the examiner by cheating on the test. If one eye has been injured, the acuity should be tested in that eye first, and the other eye must be carefully occluded. Often several pieces of tissue paper must be taped over the good eye to prevent the child from tilting the head enough to see past the occluder. With small children, a parent may be better able to keep the eye covered without upsetting the child.

b. Evaluation of the Pupils

Careful evaluation of the pupils in accident cases may help in a general appraisal of the patient's illness and in decisions regarding disposition to consultants. The pupils can be very helpful in evaluating patients with altered states of consciousness but can be interpreted only after considering the many possible reasons for abnormal pupillary size and reactivity (Table 1–4). Useful information can be gained from the swinging flashlight test in the detection of afferent pupillary defects, especially from optic nerve lesions (Marcus Gunn pupil).

Both the direct and consensual pupillary responses must be tested. When one of the pupils cannot be tested directly because it is obscured

Table 1–4. CAUSES OF ASYMMETRY OF PUPILS

1. Antecedent causes of unequal pupils.
2. Traumatic mydriasis or miosis from direct blow to the eye.
3. Iridodialysis or rupture of iris sphincter.
4. Unilateral use of topical drugs.
5. Intraorbital trauma to ciliary nerves or ganglia.
6. Horner's syndrome.
7. Intracranial third-nerve palsy.

by hemorrhage or has been injured, the consensual response will be an important indicator of the viability of the afferent visual system.

The pupils are examined in a darkened room. The initial size of each pupil is noted as well as the amount of reaction to a bright light (commonly described as 1[+], 2[+], etc. or as the resulting pupillary size). The swinging flashlight test is then performed by shining the light in one eye for four seconds and then quickly swinging it to the other eye. The examiner notes whether the pupil quickly constricts and then slowly dilates (the normal response) or merely slowly dilates (the abnormal response). When one pupil dilates relatively faster than the other, this indicates an abnormality with the afferent pathways in the eye with the more quickly dilating pupil. The afferent pupillary defect may be quantified using neutral density filters.[1] The consensual response is tested by illuminating one pupil from the side with just enough light to be able to see its response. A bright light is then shined on the other pupil while regarding the first pupil. The normal response is for the dimly illuminated pupil to react when the other pupil is illuminated.

The fixed, dilated pupil occasionally offers a diagnostic dilemma. Possibilities include impairment of the effector muscles in the eye, defective parasympathetic innervation, and the presence of atropinic substances in the eye. Pharmacologic blockage can usually be identified by the pupil's failure to constrict after administration of dilute pilocarpine.[2] Direct trauma to the iris sphincter or dilator can cause ipsilateral miosis or mydriasis (see Table 1–4). Therefore, dilatation of one pupil does not necessarily indicate the presence of a traumatically induced increase in intracranial pressure (with compression of the oculomotor nerve). On the other hand, a fixed, dilated pupil observed soon after head trauma may indicate direct nerve injury such as laceration of the oculomotor nerve or damage to its nucleus. If the pupillary dilatation occurs some time after the traumatic incident, it may indicate a subdural hematoma or some other factor leading to increased intracranial pressure and early herniation. In the case of direct trauma to the oculomotor nerve or its nucleus, the pupillary dilatation is often associated with other manifestations of oculomotor paresis, such as ptosis or extraocular muscle imbalance. In the case of generalized increased intracranial pressure as the cause of third-nerve paresis, only the pupillary fibers of the oculomotor nerve are typically involved.

Immediately after blunt trauma to the eye, a common finding is spastic constriction of the pupil associated with increased accommodation. This is generally temporary, giving way to paralytic mydriasis within a matter of minutes or several hours. At times, traumatic uveitis will ensue, and the pupil will remain small. On the other hand, direct trauma to the eye may cause tears in the pupillary sphincter, preventing the pupil from ever fully constricting.

Post-traumatic paralytic mydriasis is often permanent to some degree; associated with the pupillary abnormality is some weakness in accommodation. The response to 2% pilocarpine differentiates this pupillary abnormality from one produced by instillation of cycloplegic drops. In a pupil previously paralyzed with drugs, 2% pilocarpine will not cause *prompt* constriction, whereas pilocarpine *will* cause prompt constriction of the traumatically dilated pupil or the dilated and fixed pupil of an individual with rising intracranial pressure and third-nerve involvement.[3]

After blunt direct trauma, the eye can also mimic Horner's syndrome of sympathetic paresis owing to the common findings of miosis, ptosis, slight hyperemia of the globe, pseudoenophthalmos, and possibly a slight decrease in intraocular pressure. Anhidrosis, of course, is not related to direct ocular trauma. One of the best screening tests for oculosympathetic paresis is administration of 4% cocaine drops. When the response is positive, the pupil of the affected eye either fails to dilate or dilates less extensively than the normal pupil, which serves as the control. Before the cocaine test can be considered positive, a 2 mm difference in diameter must exist between the two pupils at the end of the test.[3]

References

1. Thompson HS, et al: How to measure the relative afferent pupillary defect. Surv Ophthalmol 26:39–42, 1981.
2. Thompson HS, Newsome DA, Loewenfeld IE: The fixed dilated pupil: sudden iridoplegia or mydriatic drops? A simple diagnostic test. Arch Ophthalmol 86:21–27, 1971.
3. McCrary J A III: *Pediatric Oculo-Neural Diseases: Case Studies.* Flushing, NY, Medical Examination Publishing Co, 1973.

2

Injuries of the Lids

2.1 BASIC CONSIDERATIONS

The first step in caring for an injury of the lid is determining the extent of the injury, with particular attention to the underlying globe. Small lacerations of the lid should be gently probed and at times explored; large ones should be laid open.

As with the management of severe burns, prophylactic antibiotics and tetanus immunization should be considered from the time of initial management. Simple, clean lid lacerations rarely develop wound infections, and the treatment of these injuries with systemic antibiotics is not justified. On the other hand, in instances of delayed repair, extensive necrotic tissue, and human bites, consideration should be given to the possibility of infection with anaerobic organisms. The use of antibiotics and tetanus prophylaxis is covered in Chapter 9.

For lacerations of the lid, the surgeon should perform a meticulous primary repair using instruments and sutures suitable to the delicacy of the task. Primary repair often produces an excellent final result after a year or more of gradual improvement. Therefore, many months should elapse before cosmetic correction of residual deformities is undertaken. Permanent deformity of the eyelids is not only detrimental to function of the eye, but the cosmetic defect also may be severely damaging to the patient's self-image. Surely, few other areas of the body require more careful reapproximation of tissue planes and precise reconstruction of defects to assure satisfactory functional and cosmetic results. However, reconstructive surgery is scarcely so well rewarded, for the rich blood supply of the eyelids, the thinness and laxity of the lid skin, and the infrequency of infection all contribute to making the tissue ideal for plastic refurbishing.

2.2 SURGICAL ANATOMY OF THE EYELIDS

A comprehensive review of lid anatomy cannot be included here, but selected features of particular importance in surgical repairs will be mentioned. The lids should be regarded as triple-layered structures: the anterior layer is composed of the skin, the middle layer is composed of the orbicularis muscle, and the posterior layer is composed of the tarsus and palpebral conjunctiva (Figure 2–1). Examination of the lid margins reveals a faint linear demarcation between the skin and conjunctiva: the "gray line" and mucocutaneous junction.

Each of the three surgical layers of the lid should be closed separately

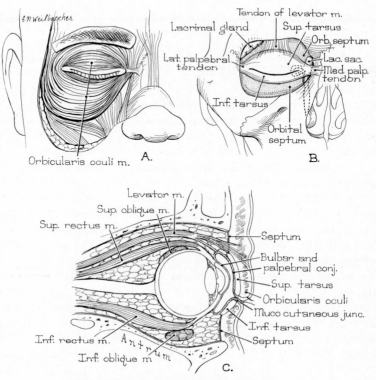

Figure 2–1. Anatomy of the lids and orbit.

in all lid lacerations that transect the tarsus. In past years, it was common practice to split the eyelids along the gray line to provide a sliding flap of skin and superficial muscle to fill a post-traumatic lid defect. Such gray-line incisions are now infrequent for that purpose, although sliding skin flaps are important reparative techniques, as will be discussed later. Because of the abundance of skin in the vicinity of the lids, large skin defects can usually be closed by undermining and sliding skin over the relatively fixed posterior layer. When there is an actual defect caused by loss of tissue from the posterior layer, the flaps must consist of tarsal tissue. These flaps must be so designed that both upper and lower lids will have a continuous margin of tarsus to maintain normal lid conformity.

The conjunctiva is a mucous membrane that covers the entire posterior surface of the lids, reaching from canthus to canthus and fornix to fornix, forming a sac that is open anteriorly at the lid fissure and closed at the limbus (see Figure 2–1). The conjunctiva is a distinct tissue layer except where it is firmly adherent to the tarsus of the lids. The loose folds of its generous recesses (the upper and lower fornices) permit marked lid and eye mobility. Like the skin of the lids, the conjunctiva has a natural laxity that permits extensive mobilization for surgical repairs such as construction of sliding tarsal flaps. As is true of other mucous membranes, the mucocutaneous junctions of the conjunctiva are abrupt, forming smooth boundaries that cannot be emulated by surgical apposition of conjunctiva to skin. Consequently, it is important to salvage as much natural lid margin as possible in lid reconstructions. Mucous membrane grafts within the conjunctival sac do exceptionally well. Usually, the grafts are taken from the contralateral eye or the buccal cavity. Skin grafts to the conjunctiva are contraindicated because of the irritating keratin debris that results. This is usually true even when the eye has been enucleated and the surgery is being performed on an anophthalmic socket.

The tarsal "plates" provide strength and curvature to the lids. The tarsi are composed of dense fibrous tissue (not cartilage) containing the meibomian glands, whose orifices are posterior to the gray line. Peripheral to the tarsi is the orbital septum, a relatively inelastic sheet of fibrous tissue (see Putterman and Urist[1] for a more detailed description). The orbital septum attaches to the periosteum at the orbital rim throughout its circumference and forms the barrier between the orbital contents and the more superficial layers of muscle and skin. *If a lid laceration contains fat, the examiner knows that the orbital septum has been perforated* (Figure 2–2). If a perforating instrument or foreign body has penetrated deeply enough to pass through the orbital septum, it may well have perforated the eyeball (see Figure 2–1). Superiorly, the tendon of the levator palpebrae muscle courses from the orbital apex to the skin of the upper lid, inserting near the upper margin of the tarsus and producing the upper lid fold. Traumatic damage to the levator muscle may therefore be signaled by an absence of lid fold as well as by blepharoptosis. Lacerations involving the superior portion of the orbit, *particularly its medial third*, sometimes involve the

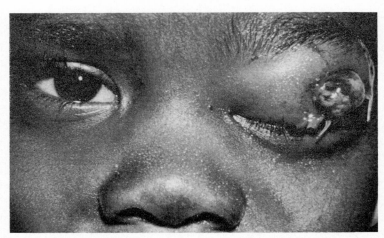

Figure 2–2. Deep laceration of left upper lid with herniation of orbital fat. In order for fat to prolapse, the orbital septum (and potentially the globe itself) must have been perforated (see Figure 2–1).

aponeurosis of the levator tendon, and they must be recognized and repaired.

That portion of the muscular layer of the eyelids overlying the tarsus inserts by means of medial and lateral tendons to the bone just within the orbital rim. In the past, these tendons have been termed the medial and lateral canthal ligaments—incorrect designations for these fibrous cords constituting muscular insertion into bone. Repair of anything but the most simple lid lacerations requires knowledge of the anatomy of the canthal tendons (see Figure 2–1).

The superficial head of the *medial* canthal tendon is short and, unlike the *lateral* canthal tendon, is infrequently damaged in trauma cases. Laterally, the pretarsal muscle inserts by a 7-mm tendon to a point just inside the lateral orbital rim; superficial to the lateral canthal tendon is a fibrous linear fascial plane, the lateral canthal raphe. It is this structure that is clamped and incised by a canthotomy, which is a means of lengthening the palpebral fissure or of relieving lid pressure on the underlying globe. Cantholysis, the sectioning of the canthal tendon often performed after canthotomy, may be necessary to decrease abnormal horizontal lid tension when lid defects are repaired by sliding flaps (see Figure 2–8). In many cases, spontaneous re-union of the severed upper or lower portions of the canthal tendon will occur, but when these tendons have been cut at the time of lid trauma, they should be identified and repaired as part of the primary surgery.

The lacrimal gland is located at the lateral aspect of the superior orbital margin (Figure 2–3). Trauma to the lacrimal gland is rare, probably because of its secluded position. Perforating injuries can lead to dacryoadenitis or can transect the ductules of the gland in the superior conjunctival cul-de-sac. Surgical anastomosis of these tiny ducts is not possible, and they must not be damaged during orbital explorations from lateral or superior approaches.

The medial portions of the eyelids contain the canaliculi of the lacrimal drainage apparatus (see Figures 2–3 and 2–17). In repair of lid lacerations, attention should be directed to the functional role of the lids—not only to the fact that complete lid closure must be obtained to protect the eye, but also to the part that the lids play in the distribution and drainage of the

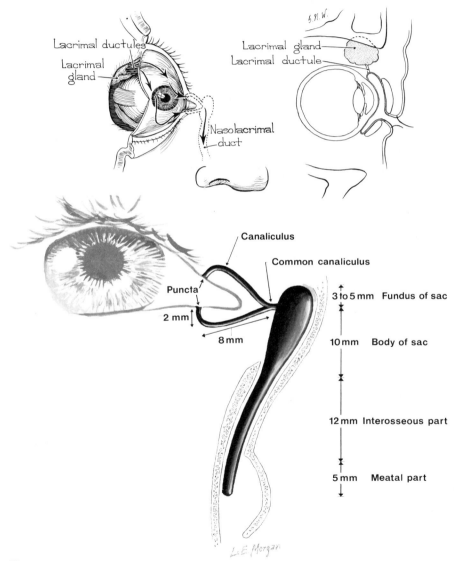

Figure 2–3. Lacrimal apparatus. (After Putterman AM: Basic oculoplastic surgery. In *Principles and Practice of Ophthalmology*. Peyman GA, Sanders D, Goldberg MF, eds; Philadelphia, WB Saunders Co, 1980, 2273.)

tears.[4] Blinking does more than moisten the cornea with tear film; the gentle squeeze of eyelid closure brings the lacrimal puncta of the lids into close contact with the pooled tear fluid of the eye, and the contraction of the orbicularis fibers assist in the propulsion of tears into the canaliculi and the lacrimal sac itself. The compression causes the tear flow to proceed into the nose via the nasolacrimal duct. The orbicularis fibers of the lower lid, in particular, should be accorded great respect at the time of injury repair; surgical skin flaps or superficial tissue deformity from primary trauma itself can cause irreversible loss of function of the lacrimal drainage passageways, even though the drainage structures themselves were spared from the original trauma.

Finally, it is useful to recall that the orbit has no lymphatics, whereas the lymphatic drainage of the eyelids is divided into two main pathways. The medial two thirds of the lids drain to the submaxillary nodes and the lateral one third to the preauricular nodes. Inflammation of the eyelids is often associated with palpable enlargement of these nodes.

2.3 ECCHYMOSES OF THE LIDS

Direct blows to the eyelids may cause ecchymoses arising from the plentiful blood supply of the lids themselves; there may be an associated orbital hemorrhage with proptosis of the eye and hemorrhage under the conjunctiva. What is on one day a unilateral "black eye" may spread to the other side in ensuing days as the blood within the lids seeps subcutaneously across the nasal bridge. An examiner should not necessarily conclude, therefore, that both orbital areas have sustained direct trauma. Blood in the lid may also gravitate to the cheek and jaw area.

Hemorrhage within the lids is of no consequence per se, but it can signal other more serious injuries to orbital contents. For example, fracture of the roof of the orbit is sometimes followed by dissemination of hemorrhage along the levator muscle, producing subconjunctival hemorrhage superiorly as well as ecchymosis of the upper lid. A ringlike distribution of periorbital blood is sometimes associated with basilar skull fracture. Orbital floor fractures may be associated with hemorrhage in the lower lid and inferior portion of the orbit. As will be described more fully later, there are also various contusion injuries within the eye that can accompany hematomas of the lids.

Treatment of lid ecchymoses is usually limited to initial cold compresses, subsequent warm compresses, and the cosmetic use of sunglasses for a fortnight.

2.4 TRAUMATIC PTOSIS

During repair of upper lid injuries, it is important to identify the levator muscle, so that the tendon can be sutured to the upper margin of the tarsus (or to its distal segment) and muscle function can be restored (see Figure 2–1).

Any upper lid swelling is associated to some degree with a drooping of the upper lid or narrowing of the lid fissure. Most often such traumatic ptosis resolves as the edema subsides and lid function returns to normal. Any persistent soreness or photophobia of the eye will produce a partial, protective ptosis that will persist as long as the irritation remains. There are times, however, when a blow to the eye is followed by a prolonged ptosis of the upper lid without evident damage to the third cranial nerve, without evident avulsion of the levator palpebrae muscle, and without abnormality of the eye. Presumably, the cause is hematoma of the muscle. Once the examiner is satisfied that there is no clinical evidence of mechanical interruption of the levator muscle, his only recourse is to wait an extended period of time before considering surgical repair. Spontaneous correction of traumatic ptosis may require a year or more. Thus, ptosis operations must not be considered until many months after blunt injury, at which time choice of repair depends on associated tissue abnormalities and degree of levator function, if any.[5]

2.5 ANIMAL AND HUMAN BITES OF THE EYELID

Bites from humans, dogs, and other animals should be allowed to heal by secondary intention after adequate debridement and extensive wound irrigation. Only with very large skin defects should primary split-thickness skin grafts be considered, but tarsorrhaphy to minimize lid deformity from contractures is a wise primary procedure if the globe itself is uninjured (Figure 2–4).

The decision to use prophylactic antibiotics must be based on the extent and age of the wound. The organisms most feared are the anaerobes and, to a lesser extent, the aerobic, gram-positive cocci. There is also the possibility of penicillinase-producing staphylococci in wounds 24 to 36 hours old. Intravenous methicillin and penicillin G would be an appropriate combination for a severe wound of this nature. For lesser infections, oral therapy might be permissible, in which case the use of cloxacillin and oral penicillin G would be appropriate. For possible gram-negative rods, the addition of gentamicin would be worthwhile. Tetanus toxoid inoculation is also an important consideration (see Table 8–2).

In the case of dog bite, prophylaxis against rabies must be considered. In any animal bite about the face or head, regardless of the health of the animal at the time of the bite, the recommendations are to begin administration of antiserum (40 IU/kg in a single intramuscular dose); there is some difference of opinion concerning whether or not the wound should be infiltrated with 500 IU of antirabies serum. If the animal is available and remains healthy for five days, then the vaccine can be discontinued. If the animal is found to be rabid or has escaped, then treatment must follow the full course (14 to 21 days).[6]

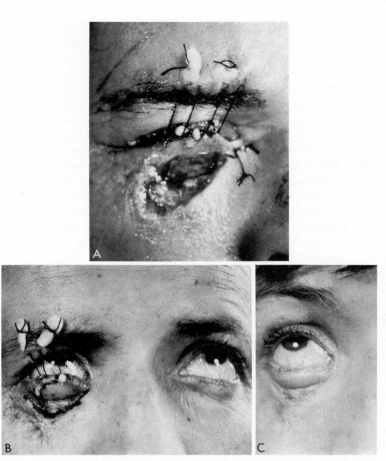

Figure 2–4. Human bite of right lower lid. (A) Initial treatment two days after the injury consisted of attachment of the avulsed lower eyelid to the medial canthal tendon region. There was a large area of skin and orbicularis muscle missing from the lower eyelid. Skin grafting was deferred owing to the late repair and the possibility of infection. The lower eyelid was placed in an elevated position for four weeks in hope that the defect would granulate spontaneously. (B) Despite this, a moderate cicatricial ectropion developed, which was repaired with a full-thickness skin graft taken from the posterior auricular area and performed two months after the injury. The lid was again elevated by suturing the lower lid margin to the eyebrow for three weeks. (C) This successfully relieved the ectropion. (This case is published through the courtesy of Allen Putterman, M.D.)

2.6 GANGRENE OF THE EYELIDS

Rarely, trauma to the eyelids initiates gangrene. This dangerous complication occurs very infrequently, undoubtedly because of the rich blood supply of the lids. However, several cases have been reported recently.[7] Physical and chemical agents lead to tissue necrosis, but a bacterial invader such as *Streptococcus* or *Proteus* produces marked pain, swelling, and redness of the affected tissues. The distended skin becomes anesthetic and turns from yellow to dark black in three to four days. Septicemia may develop. Streptococcal gangrene can be differentiated from erysipelas: patients with the latter initially have a more toxic reaction. Erysipelas does not become infected secondarily by other organisms, whereas gangrene may be complicated by the invasion of *Proteus, Pseudomonas,* and *Staphylococcus aureus.*

2.7 ANESTHESIA FOR REPAIR OF LID INJURIES

The majority of lid lacerations can be repaired under local anesthesia if the patient is cooperative. Figure 2–5 shows the customary sites of injection for those branches of the fifth and seventh cranial nerves that serve the periocular tissues. Retrobulbar anesthesia is a useful adjunct when lacerations involve the conjunctiva and when orbital hemorrhage or lacerations of the globe do not contraindicate increasing intraorbital pressure by addition of the anesthetic solution. Topical instillation anesthetics also are useful adjuncts, particularly when the effect of the injected anesthesia is waning.

Although a longer-acting local anesthetic has recently been advocated (bupivacaine), lidocaine (Xylocaine) in 2% solution is currently a favored agent for infiltration anesthesia; the addition of 2 drops of 1:1000 epinephrine per 10 ml of the anesthetic produces a more lasting effect and reduces bleeding. The amount of lidocaine injected should not exceed 500 mg (50 ml of 1% lidocaine) if used with epinephrine or 300 mg (30 ml of 1% lidocaine) if used without epinephrine. This dosage must be reduced for children and elderly or debilitated patients. Hyaluronidase is commonly

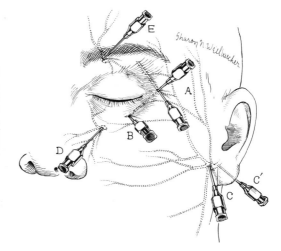

Figure 2–5. Injection points for facial and orbital anesthesia and akinesia. (A) Van Lint technique of orbicularis infiltration, (B) retrobulbar injection site, (C) O'Brien facial nerve block, (C') alternative facial nerve block by tympanomastoid fissure injection, (D) infraorbital sensory block, (E) supraorbital sensory block.

used in association with the local anesthetic. If used, the anesthetic solution should also contain epinephrine. Topical anesthetics that can be dropped onto the eye and the conjunctiva include cocaine 4%, proparacaine hydrochloride (Ophthaine) 0.5%, and others. Cocaine is probably the most effective but has the occasionally undesirable side effect of temporarily reducing corneal transparency.

Paralysis of the orbicularis muscle can be obtained by the O'Brien technique. The zygomatic arch is located and followed back to a point just above the tragus of the ear; the condyloid process of the mandible is felt to slip forward under the finger as the patient opens his mouth. The patient is directed to close his mouth, and the injection is made just anterior to the condyloid process, not in the joint itself. At this site, only 2 or 3 ml of lidocaine 2% is required for good lid akinesia (see Figure 2–5). Unlike the van Lint technique, the O'Brien method accomplishes facial muscle akinesia without increased lid swelling from the local injection. However, some local infiltration of epinephrine-fortified anesthetic solution reduces bleeding at the time of surgical repair. As shown in Figure 2–5, injections of anesthetic at the supraorbital notch and infraorbital foramen are convenient means of augmenting lid anesthesia, particularly for patients who have had no more than an O'Brien block combined with retrobulbar injection.

One advocated modification of the O'Brien technique is the injection of anesthetic solution into the tympanomastoid fissure for akinesia of the facial musculature (see Figure 2–5).[8]

The van Lint technique of akinesia and anesthesia of the eyelids employs local infiltration of the anesthetic into the deep subcutaneous tissues of the orbital margins (see Figure 2–5). As much as 10 ml of lidocaine with epinephrine added can be used in this manner. Minimal hemorrhage from the injection may occur but rarely complicates surgical repairs.

Any of the techniques for orbicularis paralysis may be used when an uncooperative patient (or one with inadvertent blepharospasm) squeezes his lids so tightly that atraumatic examination of the eye itself is otherwise impossible.

Retrobulbar injection of local anesthetic is a useful and sometimes essential adjunct to repair of lid lacerations, particularly when the bulbar conjunctiva requires surgical manipulations or when ocular motility is undesirable. Retrobulbar anesthesia should never be used with a lacerated globe; such cases require general anesthesia. Although the method of administering a retrobulbar block is relatively simple, hemorrhage, damage to the globe, and inadequate akinesia can result from improper placement of the needle. A No. 23, 35-mm Atkinson retrobulbar needle with sharp but rounded point reduces the possibility of orbital hemorrhages. After the skin has been cleansed and a wheal of anesthetic has been produced at the injection site, the patient is directed to look upward and medially. The needle is introduced through the skin just above the junction of the middle and lateral thirds of the inferior orbital margin (see Figure 2–5). The needle is passed through the orbital septum and then directed obliquely upward and slightly inward toward the apex of the orbit. The plunger is retracted to determine whether a vessel has been penetrated; if not, 1 to 3 ml of anesthetic solution is injected. It is important not to wag the needle tip, as this is the chief cause of retrobulbar hemorrhage. Some surgeons prefer to inject into the muscle cone just posterior to the globe, whereas others insert the needle further into the apex of the orbit.

A surgeon unaccustomed to lid surgery will too often forget that abrasions of corneal epithelium may occur from contact with instruments, sutures, or sponges. Undetected and unattended corneal abrasions can evolve into corneal ulcerations and create severe discomfort for the patient when the anesthetic has worn off. The use of a plastic corneal shield during lid procedures is advisable.

2.8 PREOPERATIVE PREPARATION FOR REPAIR OF LID WOUNDS

a. Eyelashes and Brow

Eyelashes may be trimmed if desired; they regrow promptly, regaining their normal length in four to six weeks. In contradistinction, the brow hair ordinarily should not be shaved, for in rare cases this hair does not regrow and at times the pattern of new brow hair is irregular. Unusual and infrequent though these misfortunes may be, the advantages of shaving the brow are slight and do not warrant the possible complications, even when the brow itself has been lacerated.

b. Cleansing the Skin and Conjunctiva

Many techniques for cleansing the skin are acceptable preoperative routines. Preliminary use of liquid green soap is time-honored. The soap (and all other antiseptic agents) should not be used within the conjunctival sac but should be applied only to the skin and the surrounding surgical field. Detergents containing iodine compounds, also used in this manner, are probably superior to soap.

Irrigation is the key to adequate wound cleansing. An intravenous set with a suspended 500-ml bottle of sterile saline solution is a convenient way to irrigate the injured region, combining lavage with tissue separation to wash away particulate foreign material. The conjunctival sac can also be thoroughly irrigated with saline, and cotton swabs ensure absence of foreign bodies in the fornices of the conjunctiva. Many surgeons follow irrigation with successive applications of tincture of iodine and isopropyl alcohol to the periocular skin.

c. Draping and Preparing for Surgery

Most patients under local anesthesia should receive intravenous fluid by slow drip in case sudden restlessness or cardiovascular distress requires intravenous medication. Use of an electrocardiographic monitor has become a standard precaution.

Draping of the wound for sterile repair depends on the site of the lesion. Cotton should be placed in the ear to prevent entrance of blood and irrigating solutions. In all cases, a head towel should be used. It is customary to employ an eye sheet with a 3- to 4-inch oval opening when only a small area of exposure is required. Adhesive plastic sheeting is a helpful means of keeping a surgical field sterile.

2.9 SIMPLE LACERATIONS OF THE LIDS

After debridement, control of bleeding, and a search for foreign bodies, the actual repair of lid lacerations is similar to wound repair elsewhere, except for the particular importance of separate-layer closure and the need for fine suture material. Prevention of contracture deformity of the lid contours is a principal concern. Poor wound closure can result in abnormally thin or thick scars and resultant impairment of lid function. Healing is usually excellent despite a patchwork of suture lines at the time of primary closure. Hawsers of 4–0 black silk have no place in repair of the lids; 6–0, 7–0, 8–0, and even 9–0 sutures made of synthetic absorbable materials, nylon, or silk are available. Proper magnification should be used as appropriate for each case; operating loupes provide visualization of the key landmarks in the surgical repair, and an operating microscope is sometimes helpful as well.

In closing a simple full-thickness laceration of the lid margin (Figure 2–6), the first sutures should reappose the landmarks of the lid margin: the squared edge of the posterior border, the gray line, and the posterior lash line. 6–0 nylon or silk sutures should be used. The initial double-armed suture is placed through the cut tarsus in the wound to exit within the squared edge at the posterior extent of the lid margin. After each side of the suture is passed, the long arms are crossed so that it can be determined if the posterior lid margin will be well apposed. The second double-armed suture is then passed through the cut tarsus in each side

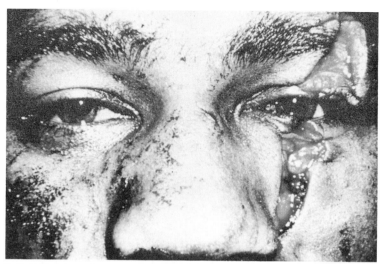

Figure 2–6. Knife injury of upper and lower lids without damage to globe. There has been no loss of tissue.

of the wound to exit through the gray line. These arms are also crossed to ensure that the lid margin is still being apposed correctly. The third suture is now passed through tarsus to exit in the posterior lash line. After these arms are crossed to check the accuracy of the apposition, the posterior, then the gray line, and finally the lash line sutures are tied. The posterior two sets of sutures are then incorporated into the knot of the lash line suture to prevent the suture ends from rubbing on the cornea. These three sutures should remain in place for two weeks.

Once the lid margin is apposed, the tarsus and skin should be closed in two layers. It is not necessary to place sutures through the conjunctiva. The tarsus can be closed with 6–0 synthetic absorbable sutures of any type. The skin and orbicularis can then be closed in one layer with 7–0 nylon or silk sutures in either a running or interrupted fashion. These sutures may be removed after four to seven days.

The lid margin sutures should not be incorporated into the knots of the skin sutures because it makes removal of the skin sutures more complicated and difficult. When dealing with children, an absorbable suture such as chromic catgut (which comes in a "mild" form for skin closure) may be used to avoid the need for suture removal.

Some simple full-thickness lacerations of the eyelids produce ragged injuries without any real loss of eyelid tissue (Figure 2–7). After debridement, the surgeon must sharpen the margins of the tarsal and skin lacerations, sacrificing as little tarsus as possible.

Many tarsal lacerations have a diagonal (rather than vertical) config-

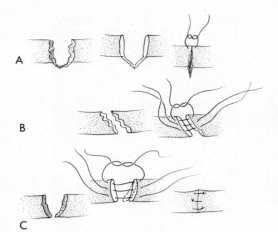

Figure 2–7. Techniques of repairing injured tarsus.

uration across the tarsus. It is not necessary to convert such lacerations into vertical or right-angle wounds if they do not involve loss of tarsal tissue. Even a beveled laceration can be repaired by accurately reapposing the severed tarsus (see Figure 2–7).

Vertical scars can result in linear contraction with notching of the eyelid margin. Thus, if the laceration is extensive, ragged, or associated with tissue loss, it is better to augment closure with a Z-plasty.[9] Hypertrophic scars are rare, particularly if the laceration is not vertical; significant keloids do not usually occur in the eyelids.

2.10 LID AVULSIONS AND LACERATIONS WITHOUT LOSS OF TISSUE

Glancing blows can avulse a lid, which then dangles free like a pedicle flap, with little or no loss of its substance (Figure 2–8). The most important factor in repair of such injuries is identification of the stump of the canthal tendon. Fractures of the orbital walls, particularly the lateral wall, can tear a tendon from its bony insertion; this possibility also must not be overlooked when the bones themselves are realigned. Such an injury is signaled by a droopy or rounded appearance of the lateral canthus and undue laxity of the lids.

The surgical approach to the canthal tendons will depend on the nature of the individual injury (Figure 2–9; see also Figure 2–8). Because lid tissues are edematous at the time of initial repair, the essential role of the canthal tendon may not be appreciated until many weeks elapse. Some lacerated tendons will reunite spontaneously if other lid tissues are restored to their proper positions, but primary repair is advisable. For an

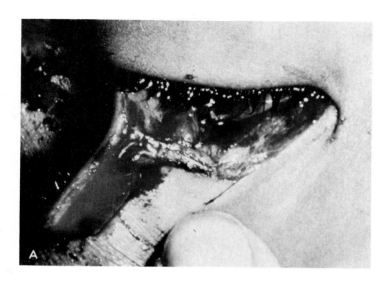

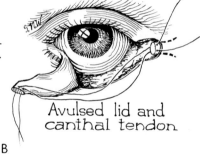

Figure 2–8. (A) Traumatic avulsion of the medial canthal tendon. (B) Demonstration of its repair.

Avulsed lid and canthal tendon

B

avulsed lid (see Figure 2–8), the tendon can be restored to its normal position (directly to the bone) with synthetic nonabsorbable suture material or fine No. 30 wire. The canthal tendon must be inserted *within* the orbital margin—not *at* the orbital margin—for proper lid conformity; avulsions of the medial canthus necessarily involve damage to the lacrimal canaliculi or sac. Repair of these structures will be discussed later.

2.11 EXTENSIVE LID LACERATIONS WITH LOSS OF TISSUE

At first glance in an emergency treatment room, the disfigurement of lid trauma can be startling (Figures 2–10 and 2–11; see also Figure 2–8): a scrambled mass of tissue with areas of unnaturally exposed eyeball, twisted lid fragments containing eyelashes displaced toward the brow, sections of exposed and everted tarsus, particles of foreign material

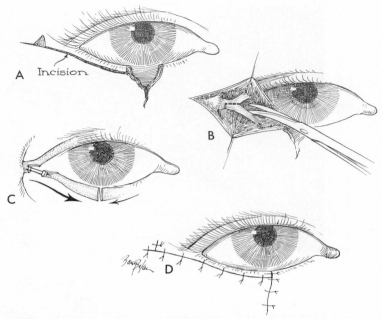

A Incision

B

C

D

Figure 2–9. Technique of cantholysis and sliding skin flap for repair of lower-lid defect. Note that the skin incision is made several millimeters below the lash margin. (A) The lateral canthal tendon is identified, and (B) a portion derived from the lower lid structure is severed and (C) recessed. (D) Subsequent closure of the tarsal defect is followed by separate closure of the undermined skin flap.

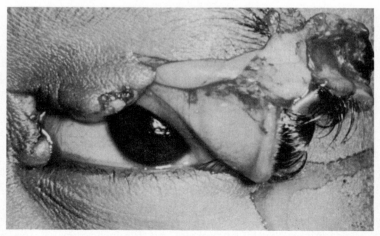

Figure 2–10. Extensively damaged upper lid without loss of tissue. This injury was caused by a dog bite.

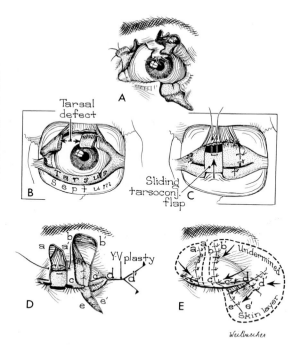

Figure 2–11. The steps necessary for repair of extensive lid lacerations. (A) Appearance of the original injury. (B) and (C) To demonstrate repair of the tarsoconjunctival layer, the skin and muscle layers have not been shown. (D) Heavy lines at the lid margins indicate where gray-line splitting has been used to assist in mobilization of tarsal flaps; the skin incisions for sliding skin flaps to fill the traumatic defects are also illustrated. (E) As in most cases of lid lacerations, the skin can be closed without use of skin grafting if sufficient mobilization of this anterior layer is accomplished.

throughout the wound, and profuse bleeding. Once the injured area has been cleansed and bleeding controlled, the pieces can usually be replaced with surprising completeness, but a logical plan of repair must be formulated. Assuming that the eye has not been injured and that x-ray films have failed to disclose a retained foreign body, the surgeon should check the integrity of the lacrimal drainage apparatus, the levator palpebrae tendon, and the orbital septum before proceeding with the repair.

Reference has already been made to the importance of suturing a severed levator tendon to the upper margin of the tarsus. The fascial layer of septum, tarsus, and canthal tendon must be organized and realigned first. Attention is then turned to the lid margins at the angles of the lid fissure. Despite extensive damage to the lateral or medial canthus, a remnant of the lid angle is usually attached to the canthal tendon, an important landmark on which to build the reconstruction. Usually, most of the tissue fragments can be drawn back into their natural positions, and denuded strips of tarsus can be salvaged. Thus, the tarsoconjunctival layer can be re-formed piecemeal by laborious tissue identification and suturing.

Primary union of a lid laceration usually is possible if one fourth or less of the lid margin is lost. Separate, sliding tarsoconjunctiva and skin flaps usually can close eyelid defects involving up to one half of the horizontal lid dimension. Only rarely are free skin grafts required, but in case they are, the surgeon should prepare a postauricular location or contralateral upper lid as a potential donor site. The use of pedicle flaps for primary repair of eyelid defects is not necessary; in fact, the cosmetic result of using a pedicle flap to replace eyelid tissue cannot compare with that of free skin grafting.

Extensive traumatic damage to eyelids should be repaired promptly (but without undue urgency) except when the surrounding tissue is acutely inflamed, edematous, or markedly ecchymotic—in which case it is wise to temporize by employing local cold applications and antibiotics, thus allowing sufficient time to permit more ideal surgical conditions.

Some basic principles in lid repair deserve review by the beginner (Table 2–1). For example, *a lid needs continuous tarsus at its margin for stability of its contour*. This is the most important principle of surgical repair of the lid and tarsus. Except for a 2- to 3-mm strip of tarsus at the lid margin, all the remaining tarsus can be sacrificed or used to fill lid tarsal defects at the lid margin. Damage to the meibomian glands is of no serious consequence.

Table 2–1. SELECTED ASSERTIONS REGARDING REPAIR OF LID LACERATIONS

Because this short text cannot include all relevant information on lid repairs, certain old and new assertions require special emphasis.

1. A lacerated tarsus must always be closed separately, using absorbable sutures, with knots on the anterior surface of the tarsus.
2. Every repaired eyelid must have a continuous strip of tarsus at the lid margin that is at least 2 to 3 mm wide.
3. Full-thickness lid lacerations should *not* be repaired by the Wheeler halving technique; direct appositional sutures using three-layer closure are recommended, although two-layer closure is conventional.
4. Never *form* a V-shaped defect in the tarsus or *close* such defects occurring by trauma; always make parallel, preferably vertical, cuts through the tarsus in fashioning sliding flaps and repairing tarsal defects.
5. Cantholysis is an important step in the repair of extensive lid defects.
6. Pedicle skin flaps (with rare exception) are not needed for eyelid reconstruction.
7. A defect involving one quarter or less of either the upper or the lower lid can be closed primarily without skin grafts. A defect involving more than one quarter and less than one half of the lid can often be closed by separate sliding tarsal flaps plus cantholysis and full-thickness skin graft.
8. Skin flaps should be mobilized not by gray-line incisions but by means of one skin incision 3 mm from the lash margin and another incision at whatever distance is necessary for undermining the full-thickness skin flap and advancing it into the lid defect.
9. Extensively burned eyelids, large lid wounds with granulation tissue, or wounds presumed to be infected should be allowed to heal by secondary intention; if necessary, healing may be aided by a thin split-thickness skin graft.
10. Vertical skin flaps can be employed for upper-lid repair but not for lower-lid repair.
11. The best donor site for full-thickness skin grafts is the postauricular skin. The upper lid is a good donor site for lower-lid reconstruction, but the reverse is not true.
12. Horizontal, linear lacerations and incisions of the skin can be closed with a running synthetic suture, whereas irregular incisions and lacerations should be closed with 8-0 or 9-0 interrupted silk sutures.
13. Silicone rubber tubing is superior to polyethylene tubing for repair of severed canaliculi.

When lacerations involve both upper and lower lids and when the globe is uninjured, a temporary tarsorrhaphy is an effective way of holding both eyelids in a good healing position. Only in such circumstances do we advise sliding tarsal flaps from the opposing eyelid to fill tarsal defects (see Figure 2–11). These vertical sliding tarsoconjunctival tongues are created by splitting of the gray line, a surgical maneuver performed far less frequently today than it was a decade ago. Gray-line splitting does produce some scarring at the mucocutaneous junction of the lid, and it can lead to unnecessary deformities of the lid margin if the surgeon is not scrupulously careful in the performance of the gray-line incision. Using loupes or an operating microscope, the surgeon and assistant grasp the lid with forceps, stretching that portion of the lid where gray-line splitting is to be performed. A knife-blade incision is made along the gray line to a depth of approximately 3 mm. Separation of the muscle layer from the tarsus is then completed for the full vertical dimension of the tarsus. A fine blunt scissors is used by spreading its blades and obtaining the plane of dissection without entry into the tarsus or the vascular orbicularis muscle (Figure 2–12). Parallel, vertical cuts are then made in the tarsus, fashioning a flap that will slide 3 to 4 mm into the tarsal defect of the opposing lid. From what has been said above, it should be clear that only the lid margins require a continuous tarsal plane. The sliding flap is secured in its recipient tarsal bed with absorbable 7–0 sutures as described for repair of simple lid lacerations.

Wounds are rarely as sharp and simple as they are in textbook diagrams. Frequently, the tarsus is raggedly torn and needs restoration of neat contours prior to closure. Yet excision of any portion of tarsus causes much greater wound stress than does comparable excision of the loose skin or muscle layers. All freshening of tarsal lacerations and defects should be done with minimal tissue sacrifice, and the parallel (not necessarily vertical) margins of tarsus must be approximated exactly.

A traumatic coloboma of the eyelid usually can be repaired by sliding

Figure 2–12. Technique for splitting the lid into an anterior layer and a posterior layer. (A) The gray-line incision is made. (B) The dissection is completed by separating the layers with blunt scissors. The posterior layer is composed of tarsus and conjunctiva; the anterior layer is composed of muscle and skin.

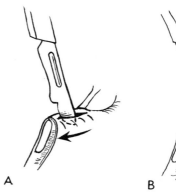

A   B

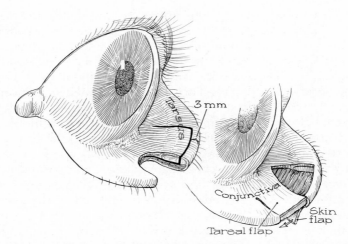

Figure 2–13. Boniuk method of tarsal defect closure by sliding tarsal flap. Note that the incision is made 3 mm posterior to the gray line and then extended vertically the full remaining width of the tarsus. The lid defect is then filled by sliding the tarsus with attached fornix conjunctiva into the defect and up to the level of the lid margin so that there is continuity of tarsus all along the repaired lid margin.

flaps if the surrounding tissue is intact and the defect has less than one half of the lid's horizontal dimension. Cantholysis, which aids in horizontal mobility of the tarsus, is usually necessary. First, a lateral canthotomy is performed with scissors at the lateral raphe but without antecedent clamping. After completion of this incision and after hemostasis has been obtained, the canthal tendon of the lid to be repaired is identified and cut (see Figure 2–9). If this maneuver to mobilize the tarsus is insufficient to permit primary closure of the defect without tightness of the tarsal or skin and muscle planes, then a sliding tarsoconjunctival flap should be used,[10] as shown in Figure 2–13. An incision is made through conjunctiva and tarsus 2 to 3 mm from the everted lid margin and parallel to the margin. To minimize tension on the wound the length of the incision should extend several millimeters beyond the defect. A vertical incision is made through the conjunctiva and tarsus and is extended through the conjunctiva into the fornix. The tarsoconjunctival flap is undermined from the overlying orbicularis muscle, and the conjunctiva is undermined into the fornix. The mobilized flap is then slid into the area of the defect, and 6–0 chromic catgut sutures are used to approximate the edges of the flap at the lid margin. Management of the skin defect will be discussed hereafter.

Once the posterior surgical layer of tarsus and conjunctiva has been reconstructed by securing any avulsed canthal tendon, suturing orbital septal defects, and repairing the tarsus itself, the muscle and skin layers are closed separately. There is marked variation among individuals in the laxity of both skin and muscle, with slackness more pronounced in the

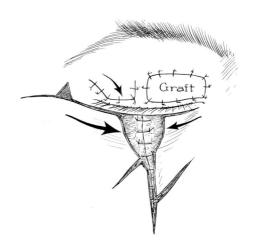

Figure 2–14. Technique for repair of lower lid. Skin defects of the lower lid should be closed by horizontal sliding flaps, with skin mobilized from the temporal portion of the lower lid and lateral canthal area; vertical skin flaps can be used for closing defects of the upper lid when available skin is abundant; large skin defects, as shown in the upper lid medially, require full-thickness skin grafts.

elderly. Superficial muscle fibers are closely related to the skin layer, and there is no true plane for dissection of skin from muscle, yet pretarsal muscle should be repaired separately and should not be mobilized as a single flap combined with the skin. The bulk of the muscle layer, no matter how torn, should be brought into continuity over the repaired tarsus.

Simple undermining of lid skin often is sufficient for mobilization and closure of tissue defects that do not include the lid margin. Commonly, however, a sliding skin flap must be employed, taking advantage of more lax and available skin from the lateral canthal region whenever possible. It is no longer recommended that sliding skin flaps be initiated by making one of the parallel incisions at the gray line. Current recommended practice consists of making the incision near the lid margin, approximately 3 mm from the lashes so that the lash follicles are not damaged. A flap of undermined skin with superficial muscle attached to it can be brought medially, with or without using auxiliary incisions, to prevent lateral skin traction (Figure 2–14). The use of Z- and Y-plasties is often of great value in repair of extensive lid defects. They represent well-known surgical maneuvers[9] and need not be discussed in detail here. Similarly, excision of small lid triangles and the prevention of dog-ears should be plastic techniques familiar to the surgeon. It is important to avoid tension on a flap; the sutures should do little more than hold the tissue margins together. The use of cantholysis therefore deserves repeated mention.

Infected tissue, granulation tissue already present, or extensive lid burns should be either allowed to heal by secondary intention or covered with a thin split-thickness graft.

2.12 SKIN GRAFTS IN PRIMARY EYELID REPAIRS

As mentioned earlier, only rare injuries to the eyelids require skin grafting at the time of primary repair. But large skin avulsions in the lid and lateral canthal areas occasionally do occur and can be repaired by the ophthalmologist familiar with basic techniques of plastic surgery.

Full-thickness skin grafts (taken from the contralateral upper lid or postauricular area) provide the best color match and do not contract postoperatively as is the case with split-thickness grafts. A word of caution: If the patient's injury is unilateral and the globe has been severely damaged, it is unwise to use the contralateral upper lid as a donor site at the time of primary repair. Not only is it psychologically undesirable from the patient's viewpoint, but any complications to the good eye that might result from taking such a graft would be most undesirable.

A useful technique for obtaining postauricular full-thickness skin is as follows. The defect to be filled by the skin graft is carefully measured, or a piece of gauze is cut to conform to its precise dimensions. An identical or only slightly larger mark is made to outline the donor area in the postauricular region with methylene blue. The donor site should be centered over the cephaloauricular angle, as this facilitates closure of the donor defect. (The defect must be closed primarily with undermined adjacent skin.) Using toothed forceps or skin hooks for traction, the full-thickness graft is excised freehand by sharp dissection. The graft is then placed in the recipient bed and secured with multiple interrupted 8-0 black silk sutures, with long arms left on the sutures so that they can be tied over a rolled piece of Telfa for four to five days.

A tight dressing over the ear must be removed within 24 hours; early removal will prevent an asymmetric ear-flattening sometimes reported with removal of large skin grafts from this area. The graft should never extend posteriorly to hair-bearing skin, for growth of hair from a graft to the eyelids is difficult to curtail in later years.

Although it is important for ophthalmologists to be familiar with split-thickness skin grafting, few will choose to undertake this work without the assistance of a specialist in soft tissue repairs.

Split-thickness skin grafts, whether cut thick or thin, promote prompt, spontaneous healing of the donor site. The closure necessitated by full-thickness excision is thus avoided. Grafts are generally cut thin for defects that are less than ideal recipient tissues: severe burns, gunshot abrasions, and involvement of eyelids that is particularly extensive. Thick split-thickness skin grafts often provide excellent tissue for large, clean defects. These grafts are best taken with a drum-type, hand-operated dermatome, often from the anterolateral part of the neck where the skin is similar in color and texture.

Split-thickness grafts must be cut considerably larger than the defect to be filled. Not only will the tissue shrink when laid on the recipient site prior to suturing, but there will be further contraction in the postoperative period and thereafter. In general, the cleaner and smaller the recipient site, the thicker the donor tissue should be. Fat should be dissected from any full-thickness graft. As a general rule, the thin upper lid is better replaced by split-thickness grafts (if not by skin from the contralateral upper lid or postauricular space), whereas the lower eyelid is less mobile and more effectively repaired by full-thickness tissue. When defects between the medial canthus and the bridge of the nose are grafted, the surgeon should be particularly careful to get good apposition of the graft to the deep underlying tissues; this is facilitated by stab incisions in the graft (to allow drainage of serosanguineous fluid) and by a postoperative dressing tightly applied for 24 to 48 hours. The dressing must never exert direct, firm pressure on the globe, for with concomitant orbital swelling and/or bleeding, a central retinal artery occlusion could result.

2.13 TRAUMATIC LOSS OF THE EYELIDS

Before the discussion of the immediate management of traumatic loss of the eyelids, a reminder may be useful: The scene of the accident should be searched for avulsed eyelids, since this tissue can be re-placed. It constitutes "donor" material more ideal than any alternative.

There is an interesting case of a child's upper lid being bitten off by a horse; the lid was found and sutured in place; it has done well except for the loss of eyelashes.[11]

In the event of almost complete loss of the eyelids, priority attention must be given to protection of the globe, which may be completely spared from the devastation that has destroyed the eyelids. Prior to the extensive plastic surgery necessary for rebuilding the eyelids, effective protection of an exposed but uninjured globe can be obtained in several ways. For short-term maintenance of necessary moisture of the eye, a piece of plastic film (Saran Wrap) can be sealed over the orbit with ophthalmic ointment at points of skin contact. This simple method may be extremely effective (see Figure 5–6). Ocular bandages of similar material are commercially available.* An alternative method utilizes the laxity of conjunctiva of the upper and lower fornix.[12] *Without any dissection*, the conjunctiva can be grasped at the upper fornix with forceps and a suture passed through it and brought through a similar fold from the lower fornix in the same vertical line. Thus, by using multiple interrupted sutures, a double thickness of conjunctiva can be brought over the globe, and a horizontal straight-line closure of conjunctiva across the cornea can be obtained

---

*Procedure Medical Products, Ltd., New York, New York.

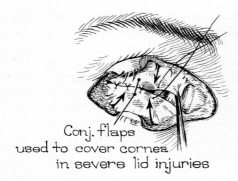

Conj. flaps
used to cover cornea
in severe lid injuries

Figure 2–15. Temporary globe protection. A double thickness of bulbar and fornix conjunctiva may be used for temporary protection of the globe with injuries involving loss of the lids. This method does not require dissection. Separation of the approximated tissue will occur within a few days. Soft (hydrophilic) lenses are not good substitutes, for such protection against exposure is exceedingly temporary and is complicated by drying of the lens and damage to the cornea, if not extrusion of the lens, when there is marked loss of the lids.

(Figure 2–15). These sutures will not hold for more than a few days, but this is more than enough time to plan the plastic revision of the lids. For long-term protection of the eye, a thin (dissected) conjunctival hood flap can be brought down over the cornea and will remain until surgically removed.[13]

Rebuilding a lid often requires sliding flaps, mucous membrane grafts, and even composite autografts, the details of which are not appropriate to a short text of this nature. Readers can refer to authoritative sources.[3, 9, 14–18] A technique of composite grafting[19] (full-thickness lid with skin, muscle, and tarsus) from the contralateral lower lid has much merit, but the occasional lid surgeon is urged to refer cases of that nature to specialists.

2.14 INJURIES OF THE LACRIMAL APPARATUS

a. Diagnosis

The anatomy of the lacrimal drainage apparatus is illustrated in Figure 2–3. Because injury to the lacrimal apparatus usually produces gross abnormalities of the tissue or obvious functional disturbances, sensitive tests of drainage function[20] are not often required for emergency room diagnosis. Lacerations within the medial fourth of the lids may impair tear drainage to the nose by direct injury to the puncta, the canaliculi, the lacrimal sac, or the nasolacrimal duct. If there is any doubt that the lacrimal system has been invaded, saline can be gently irrigated through the puncta and the patient asked if the liquid can be felt in the back of the throat.

Lid injuries may also disrupt lacrimal drainage indirectly if lid deformity causes poor pumping by the orbicularis muscle or poor apposition of the punctum against the eyeball. In repair of such lid lacerations, attention must be directed to the normal conformity of the lid as well as to the severed canaliculus.

b. Repair of Lacrimal System Injuries

Repair of a canaliculus is not always successful, but it is well worth undertaking. The closer the laceration is to the punctum, the higher the probability of successful surgical repair. Although the lower canaliculus has been said to be the most important of the two, there is no good evidence that either the upper or lower canalicular system is any more important than the other.

For surgical repair, the following procedures are employed and are most effectively accomplished with the use of an operating microscope. After instillation and injection of local anesthetic (or after placing the patient under general anesthesia if the patient is a child, is inebriated, or is otherwise uncooperative), a punctal dilator is used to widen the aperture to the canaliculus, permitting passage of probes. At times a one-snip procedure (vertical cut of the punctum with sharp scissors) is necessary if intubation is to be performed. A Bowman probe is then passed through the punctum, and the appearance of its tip in the wound identifies the distal end of the canaliculus.

The microscope is used to carefully inspect the medial edge of the wound in search of the proximal cut end of the canaliculus. The Bowman probe often can be used as a pointer to help in this identification. If the proximal end cannot be found, saline can be gently irrigated into the opposite punctum and its appearance in the wound monitored. The process of irrigation, observation, drying the wound, and reirrigation often must be repeated several times before the cut end can be found.

If it is impossible to find the proximal end of the canaliculus, the surgeon has two alternatives. First, the wound may be sutured without repair of the canaliculus. In most cases, if only one of the canaliculi has been injured, epiphora will not develop.[21, 22] The alternative is to pass a Worst pigtail probe[23] through the opposite punctum, through the lacrimal sac, and into the wound through the proximal end of the canaliculus. There are two major objections to this technique. A great deal of manipulation of the (previously) normal arm of the lacrimal system is often required and may result in injury to what is potentially the only workable canaliculus. In addition, it is often difficult to find the opening in the lacrimal sac of the opposite canaliculus. If the opening cannot be found, the repair cannot be completed.

Once the proximal end of the canaliculus has been identified, its orifice is dried and a marking pen is used to mark it. Saline is irrigated through the orifice to determine if the proximal part of the system is intact. A stent is then placed through the puncta and across the wound,

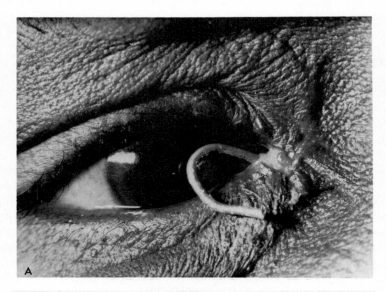

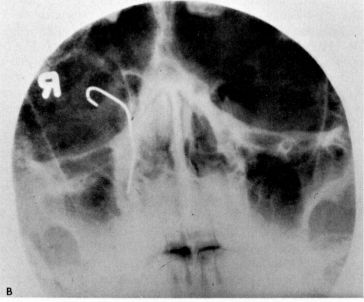

Figure 2–16. Metal-probe repair of lower canaliculus laceration. A metal probe is inserted into the nasolacrimal duct. Although the transected ends of the canaliculus were not directly sutured, they were held in close apposition by uniting the surrounding subcutaneous tissues. (A) External appearance. (B) Internal appearance. The probe should remain in position for at least eight weeks. Management of this case proved successful in that there was no epiphora, and dye placed in the conjunctival cul-de-sac and in the lower canaliculus entered the nose without difficulty. Nonetheless, direct suturing of the canaliculus is preferable whenever feasible.

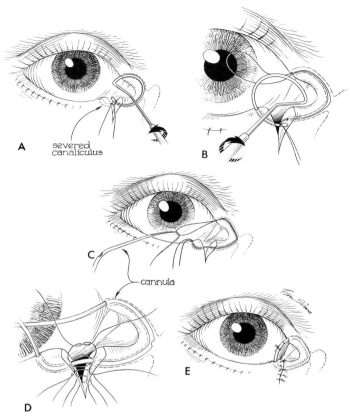

Figure 2–17. Worst's method of identifying and repairing a severed canaliculus.

and the wound is sutured as described above (see Section 2.9). The easiest stent to use is the Veirs[24, 25] rod. This consists of a small metal rod swedged to a 4–0 silk suture. The rod is simply inserted until it bridges the wound, and the suture is ultimately incorporated into a suture in the cheek (Figure 2–16). The stent should remain in place for six weeks to two months.

Another stent is Silastic tubing, which is available from several manufacturers and usually comes swedged to long metal rods similar to Bowman probes. Several techniques have been described. A long piece of tubing can be passed through the wound, similar to the manner in which the Veirs rod is used, and the external end of the tube sutured onto the skin. The metal probes may be passed through the upper and lower systems and retrieved in the nose. The probes are then cut off of the tubes and the Silastic is tied together. Finally, if the pigtail probe is used, the Silastic can be tied so that the tube connects the upper punctum to the lower, with a knot in the lacrimal sac (Figure 2–17). In each case, the Silastic tube should be left in as long as possible, but at least for six weeks.

Lacerations involving both the upper and lower puncta require an attempt to repair both canaliculi, as it is not certain whether either repair will be successful. The laceration may also involve the lacrimal sac, in which case a dacryocystorhinostomy may be necessary. There is no evidence that such a repair should be done at the time of the initial surgery, especially since not all patients with such injuries will end up with symptomatic epiphora.[22]

References

1. Putterman AM, Urist MJ: Surgical anatomy of the orbital septum. Ann Ophthalmol 6:290–294, 1974.
2. Callahan A: Surgery of the Eye. Vol. I, Injuries. Springfield, Ill, Charles C Thomas Co, 1950.
3. Callahan A: Reconstructive Surgery of the Eyelids and Ocular Adnexa. Birmingham, Ala, Aesculapium Publishing Co, 1966.
4. Jones LT: An anatomical approach to problems of the eyelids and lacrimal apparatus. Arch Ophthalmol 66:111–124, 1961.
5. Berke RN: Surgical treatment of traumatic blepharoptosis. Am J Ophthalmol 72:691–698, 1971.
6. Conn HF (ed): Current Therapy 1974. Philadelphia, W B Saunders Co, 1974.
7. Ross J, Kohlehepp PA: Gangrene of the eyelids. Ann Ophthalmol 5:84–88, 1973.
8. Haik GM, Coles WH, McFetridge EM: Intraocular Injuries: Their Immediate Surgical Management. Philadelphia, Lea & Febiger, 1972.
9. Smith B, Cherubini TD: Oculoplastic Surgery. St. Louis, C. V. Mosby Co, 1970, 61–70.
10. Boniuk M: Lid reconstruction with swinging tarsconjunctival flaps from the same lid: a new technique. In press.
11. Iliff CE: Personal communication.
12. Haik GM: A fornix conjunctival flap as a substitute for the dissected conjunctival flap: a clinical and experimental study. Trans Am Ophthalmol Soc 52:497–524, 1954.
13. Gundersen T: Conjunctival flaps in the treatment of corneal disease with reference to a new technique of application. Arch Ophthalmol 60:880–888, 1958.
14. Cutler NL, Beard C: A method for partial and total upper lid reconstruction. Am J Ophthalmol 39:1–7, 1955.
15. Frueh BR; A method for reconstruction of the lower eyelid. Am J Ophthalmol 75:710–712, 1973.
16. Hughes WL: Ophthalmic Plastic Surgery: A Manual Prepared for the Use of Graduates in Medicine (Second Edition). Rochester, Minn, American Academy of Ophthalmology and Otolaryngology, 1964.
17. King JH Jr, Wadsworth JAC: An Atlas of Ophthalmic Surgery (Second Edition). Philadelphia, J B Lippincott Co, 1970.
18. Mustarde JC, Jones LT, Callahan A: Ophthalmic Plastic Surgery—Up-to-Date. Birmingham, Ala, Aesculapium Publishing Co, 1970.
19. Youens WT, Westphal C, Barfield FT, Youens HT Jr: Full thickness lower lid transplant. Arch Ophthalmol 77:226–229, 1967.
20. Putterman AM; Evaluation of the lacrimal system. Eye Ear Nose Throat Monthly 51:212–216, 1972.
21. Saunders DH, Shannon GM, Flanagan JC: The effectiveness of the pigtail probe method of repairing canalicular lacerations. Ophthalmic Surg 9(3):33–40, 1978.
22. Canavan UM, Archer DB: Long-term review of injuries to the lacrimal drainage apparatus. Trans Ophthalmol Soc UK 99:201–204, 1979.
23. Worst JGF: Method for reconstructing torn lacrimal canaliculus. Am J Ophthalmol 53:520–522, 1962.
24. Veirs ER: Malleable rods for immediate repair of the traumatically severed lacrimal canaliculus. Trans Am Acad Ophthalmol Otolaryngol 66:263–264, 1962.
25. Veirs ER; The Lacrimal System: Proceedings of the First International Symposium. St. Louis, C. V. Mosby Co, 1971.

Fractures of the Orbit

Orbital trauma is typically signaled by ecchymosis and lid swelling of a moderate to severe degree, by mild to severe proptosis, and by ophthalmoplegia from hemorrhage within the orbit. In addition, there may be subcutaneous emphysema (crepitus palpable through the lids) from fractures of sinuses and localized anesthesia of the skin in areas innervated by the supraorbital and infraorbital branches of the trigeminal nerve. Defects in the orbital rim can sometimes be palpated, even when the skin is edematous.

A variety of injuries may occur following blunt trauma to the orbit. While many of these potential injuries are covered in Chapter 11, this chapter will deal with fractures of the orbital bones.

Fractures sometimes cannot be diagnosed until special x-ray views are obtained, but they are suggested by a variety of clinical signs. For example, fractures of the roof of the orbit are often followed by hemorrhage into the upper lid and subconjunctival hemorrhage on the lateral aspect of the globe. Cerebrospinal fluid rhinorrhea may also be associated with orbital roof fractures. Lateral wall fractures are more apt than other orbital fractures to be associated with avulsion of the optic nerve and profound loss of vision. Medial wall fractures usually produce orbital

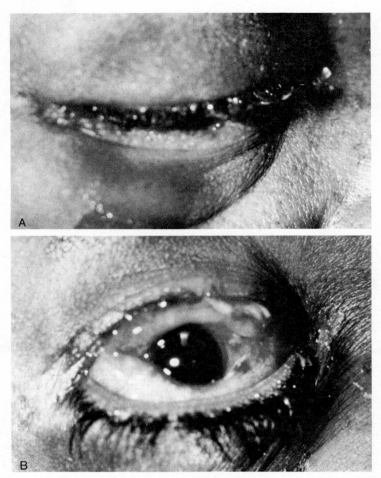

Figure 3–1. Subconjunctival emphysema after a medial orbital wall fracture. (A) The patient's appearance at rest. (B) With the eyelid retracted, erythema and chemosis are apparent.

Illustration continued on opposite page

emphysema, which, even if not palpable, is frequently visible on x-ray films. Systemic antibiotics are indicated when paranasal sinuses are fractured, but surgical repair is not necessarily undertaken if there is no damage to the orbital contents. The patient must avoid nose blowing or muscular straining if an orbital fracture into one of the sinuses is suspected; otherwise, sudden inflation of the orbit and proptosis may result (Figure 3–1).

The percentage of accurate diagnosis of orbital fractures is greatly increased by well-planned, technically excellent x-rays. The proper use of radiologic studies is described in Chapter 6.

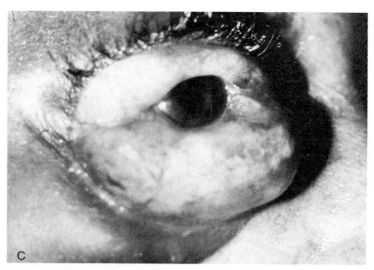

Figure 3–1. *Continued.* (C) After a spontaneous sneeze, marked subconjunctival emphysema appears. The air disappeared over a period of 20 minutes.

3.1 BLOW-OUT FRACTURES OF THE ORBITAL FLOOR

When the force of a blunt object (such as a fist or baseball) is exerted on the orbit, there is compression of orbital tissues; the markedly increased hydraulic pressure within the orbit may result in a blow-out at the site of the weakest portion of the orbit, the floor. This is especially true if the trauma is to the inferolateral aspect of the orbit.[1] Orbital fat may prolapse into the maxillary antrum, and the inferior rectus and inferior oblique muscles are often either included with or restrained by the incarcerated tissues (Figures 3–2 and 3–3). When these two ocular muscles are caught in the incarceration, not only is their function restricted but they also serve as limiting bands that prevent full-range contraction of other ocular muscles not involved in the fracture. As a result, downward gaze may be reduced because of a pinched inferior rectus muscle. However, *upward gaze is often more impaired.* This occurs not only because of incarceration of or damage to the inferior oblique muscle but also because the superior rectus cannot elevate the globe against the short rein of the trapped inferior rectus.

Definitive diagnosis of orbital floor fracture is not necessary at the time of emergency room examination; other injuries may take precedence, and the surgeon often must wait several days for orbital swelling to subside enough to permit adequate clinical examination. A blow-out fracture is never an emergency, whereas simultaneously incurred globe injuries frequently are.

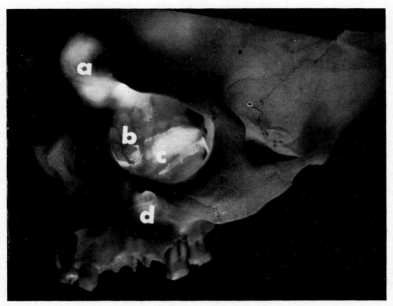

Figure 3–2. Illumination within the sinuses of a human skull. (a) The frontal sinus, (b) the ethmoid sinuses, (c) the thin orbital floor, (d) the maxillary antrum.

Clinical suspicion of a blow-out fracture is based on one or more of the following findings: anesthesia of the ipsilateral side of the nose and the skin of the lower lid; diplopia from limitation of the inferior rectus and inferior oblique muscles (Figures 3–4, 3–5, and 3–6); pain of the

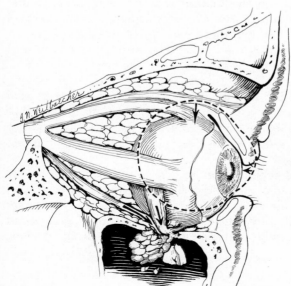

Figure 3–3. Blow-out fracture of the orbital floor. The dotted line indicates the normal position of the globe. The inferior oblique and inferior rectus muscles are restrained by the incarcerated orbital tissues.

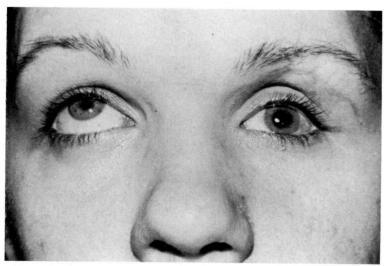

Figure 3–4. Old blow-out fracture of the left orbit with enophthalmos and limited upward gaze of the left eye.

affected side on upward gaze; positive forced-duction test; and downward and inward displacement of the globe with increase in the supratarsal sulcus (see Figure 3–4), occurring several weeks after injury when orbital swelling has resolved.

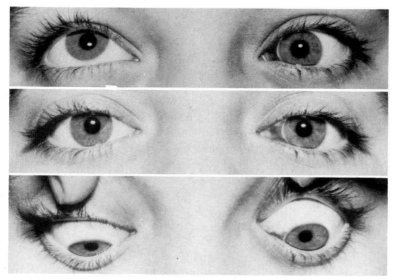

Figure 3–5. Fresh blow-out fracture of left orbit with limitation of upward and downward movement of the left eye.

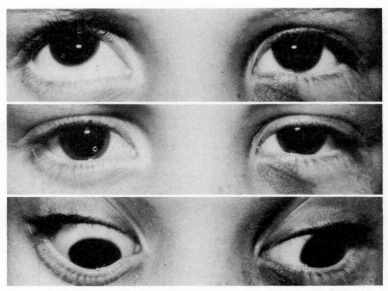

Figure 3–6. Following blow-out fracture, the physical signs are similar to those shown in Figure 3–5.

a. The Forced-duction Test

When upward gaze is impaired after trauma, it is helpful to determine the type of injury by the *forced-duction test*, which helps in differentiating limitation of motion due to orbital edema, muscle contusion, and nerve damage from limitation caused by incarceration of the inferior muscles in a floor fracture site.

After topical anesthesia, a toothed forceps is used to grasp both the conjunctiva and Tenon's fascia (at the insertion of the inferior rectus muscle, about 7 mm below the limbus). The patient is asked to look up, and the examiner rotates the eye upward; if there is a full range of motion, there is no physical entrapment of periocular tissues in a fracture site, and limitation of voluntary supraduction may be explained on the basis of such causes as true paresis of the superior rectus or inferior oblique muscle. The contralateral eye may be compared as to the resistance encountered in each direction of gaze.

If the affected eye does not elevate even with manual force, something is restraining the eye—usually the incarceration of tissue in an orbital floor fracture. A positive test, in which definitely increased resistance is encountered, virtually confirms the diagnosis of blow-out fracture with incarcerated orbital tissues.

Of course, the forced-duction test can be used to test the motility of the other rectus muscles as well. In addition, the test may be positive in cases of dysthyroid myositis and in the superior oblique tendon sheath syndrome (Brown's syndrome). When doing forced ductions, the inexperienced examiner should not mistake posterior displacement of the eyeball for improved ocular motility.

Because of lid swelling and the discomfort of forced motility, the forced-duction test is not always practical for emergency room diagnosis.

b. Computerized Tomography in Blow-out Fractures

Recent studies have demonstrated the usefulness of computerized tomography in the diagnosis and management of blow-out fractures.[2] Specifically, patients in whom muscle tissue trapped within the maxillary antrum can be seen in the coronal CT scan are most likely to develop intractable diplopia. Likewise, orbital expansion seen on the coronal CT scan correlates with subsequent development of enophthalmos. Future prospective study will be necessary to substantiate these data.

c. Indications for Repair of Blow-out Fractures

In orbital blow-out fractures, the indications for surgery are not always clear-cut. It would appear that a fracture, in the absence of significant physical signs or symptoms, does *not* invariably require operative intervention.[3-7] Significant, cosmetically unacceptable enophthalmos and disabling diplopia are the most obvious indications for exploration. Conversely, should these not be present and should the patient be visually asymptomatic, the necessity for surgical repair has not yet been clearly substantiated. The incidence of pathologic sequelae in untreated fractures that are initially asymptomatic is extremely low.[5, 7, 8]

If the patient has clear-cut signs of an orbital blow-out fracture accompanied by a severe degree of permanent loss of vision (secondary to a macular choroidal rupture or unrepaired macular retinal detachment), repair of the floor fracture is probably not justified unless there is marked enophthalmos or unless the initial examination provides evidence of a large incarceration. If no surgery is performed, the patient will never be bothered by diplopia because of the absence of binocular vision.

Other intraocular concomitants of blow-out fracture of the orbit that render surgical exploration of the orbital floor superfluous include central retinal artery occlusion and penetrating injury. Pressure on the globe created in exposing the orbital floor is sufficient that the coexistence of a penetrating injury is usually a contraindication to orbital floor repair immediately after injury and within several weeks thereafter. Other ocular injuries, such as a dislocated lens, vitreous hemorrhage, or macular edema, must be assessed individually, since many eyes traumatized in these ways can recover normal vision. Moreover, if the cosmetic defect seems excessive, there is some justification for surgical repair even if the prognosis for vision is relatively poor.

In summary, the basic indications for repairing an orbital floor fracture are the prevention of subsequent subjective diplopia and the prevention of cosmetically significant enophthalmos. Should these goals be irrelevant to the condition of an individual patient or should serious ocular injury coexist, surgical repair of the fracture is rarely justified. If they persist or occur subsequently, both diplopia and enophthalmos can be treated by techniques unrelated to floor fracture repair such as prisms, strabismus surgery, or oculoplastic surgery.

d. Timing of Surgery

Exploration of the orbital floor should never be considered an emergency measure. Surgery can safely be delayed for up to 14 days without risking irreversible scarring and fibrosis. Patients who initially have no diplopia or who lose the diplopia within 14 days of the injury need not undergo surgery at all, unless x-ray films show extensive defects in the orbital floor that could cause marked enophthalmos if not repaired. Surgery under emergency conditions is not justified unless the patient is undergoing a necessary operation for other, simultaneously incurred, facial trauma.

Conversely, neglected cases can be effectively operated on despite a three- to four-week interval after trauma. However, repair in such cases becomes technically more difficult, and the results are more uncertain owing to inflammatory and reparative processes in the injured tissues. Despite these hindrances, successful results have been achieved, even when the surgery was performed months and even years after the initial trauma.

3.2 SURGICAL REPAIR OF BLOW-OUT FRACTURES

a. Anesthesia and Sterile Draping

Exploration of the orbital floor is best performed with the patient under general anesthesia, although local anesthesia can be used if necessary. The anesthetist should realize that the surgeon may wish to inject epinephrine into the lid to decrease operative bleeding. A transoral approach to the maxillary antrum may be required, and therefore a cuffed endotracheal or nasotracheal tube rotated to the opposite side of the patient's face should be used. Even with the exploration of the maxillary antrum, there is rarely enough blood loss to require transfusion. However, such a need occasionally does arise.

Surgical preparation of the conjunctival sac and the skin is performed in the routine fashion and should include the entire face and mandible.

The sterile draping should be performed in a way that will allow a transoral approach to the maxillary sinus if the surgeon subsequently chooses to employ it.

b. Forced Ductions

After prepping and draping the patient, the forced ductions of the injured eye should be reassessed and the degree of resistance compared with that on the uninjured side (Figure 3–7:1). A 4-0 silk suture for subsequent use during the extrication of incarcerated tissues should be passed under the insertion of the inferior rectus muscle and kept in this position throughout the operation (Figure 3–7:2). The suture can then be used whenever the forced ductions are to be retested, thus preventing repeated trauma to the conjunctiva and subconjunctival tissues.

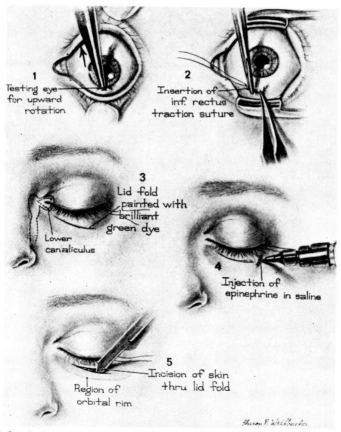

Figure 3–7. Surgical technique of orbital blow-out fracture repair. (Drawing previously published and reproduced by permission from Goldberg MF: Surgical repair of orbital blow-out fractures. In *Diagnosis and Management of Blow-out Fractures of the Orbit, with Clinical, Radiological, and Surgical Aspects.* Milauskas AT, ed; Springfield, Ill, Charles C Thomas, 1969.)

Illustration continued on following page

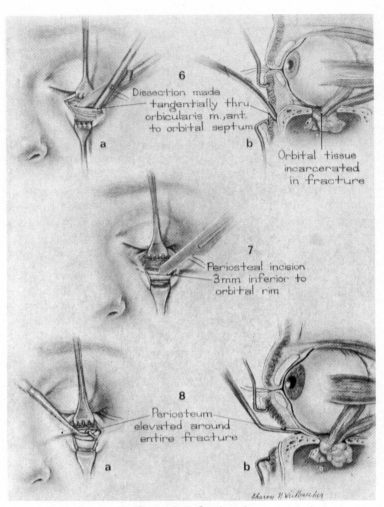

Figure 3–7. *Continued.*

Illustration continued on opposite page

c. Types of Skin Incisions

Three general types of skin incisions are employed in blow-out fracture surgery.

Lash Margin Incision. A lash margin incision is made through skin only, 1 or 2 mm inferior to the lash margin, for the length of the lower lid. The advantage of this incision is its great cosmetic acceptability; in general, the scar becomes invisible. After the skin incision, dissection is carried inferiorly to the level of the inferior orbital rim, raising a skin flap.

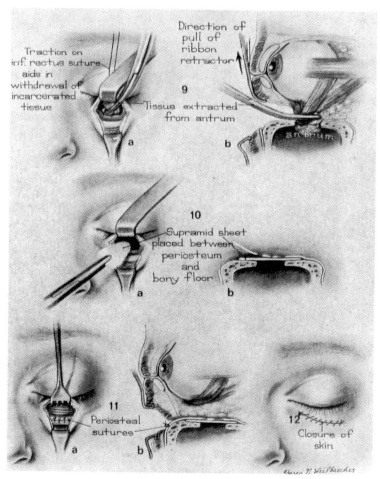

Figure 3–7. *Continued.*

The subcutaneous tissues are then separated until the orbital rim is exposed. Raising the skin flap constitutes the most important disadvantage of the lash margin incision, since the dissection is technically tedious and time-consuming and inadvertent production of a cutaneous buttonhole is always a possibility. Furthermore, good exposure of the orbital floor is somewhat more difficult to obtain with a lash margin incision than with other types of incisions.

Inferior Orbital Rim Incision. The approach by way of the inferior orbital rim is technically the easiest. In one stroke, a curvilinear incision corresponding to the shape of the inferior orbital rim is made through skin and subcutaneous tissues down to the inferior orbital rim. Minimal subcutaneous dissection is required, as the periosteum of the inferior orbital rim lies rather close to the skin in this location. However, this incision provides the least satisfactory cosmetic result, as there is frequently no natural skin fold at this position. Furthermore, the cutaneous scar often becomes involved in the immediately underlying periosteal scar, with subcutaneous fibrosis and retraction. Thus, the chance of developing a cosmetically disfiguring scar, with or without ectropion, is greater with this incision than with either of the other approaches.

Lower Lid Fold Incision. The approach through the lower lid employs an incision made in a curvilinear fashion in the natural fold of the lower lid, which usually lies midway between the lash margin and the inferior orbital rim. To preserve the natural skin fold, the line of the fold should be marked with a surgical pen prior to manipulating the tissue (Figure 3–7:3). The subcutaneous tissues, including the orbicularis muscle, can then be injected with a solution containing epinephrine, which will improve hemostasis. If traumatic lid edema or hemorrhage or both make the lid incision and subsequent rim exposure difficult, hyaluronidase (150 units; Wydase) can be added to the epinephrine solution. Rapid dissipation of the swelling occurs.

The incision should be made through the skin to the level of the superficial orbicularis muscle (Figure 3–7:5). The orbicularis should be split obliquely by blunt and sharp dissection with the points of small blunted scissors directed inferiorly toward the orbital rim (Figure 3–7:6). During this dissection, the surgeon should be cognizant of the location of the orbital septum, and the plane of dissection should be kept anterior to the orbital septum at all times. Should the orbital septum be perforated, there will be an immediate presentation of loose, lobulated orbital fat. No great complication ensues, but the surgeon may wish to repair the orbital septum with one or two interrupted sutures of 6-0 plain catgut. Herniation of fat through a perforated orbital septum can produce a lumpy lower lid.

In any of the skin incisions, great care should be taken with the *nasal*most end of the incision, since the inferior lacrimal canaliculus, and even the lacrimal sac, can be inadvertently lacerated (see Figure 2–3). Moreover, a downward curve of the *temporal* aspect of the incision helps to avert cutting of lymphatics, with subsequent localized lymphedema.

d. Handling the Periosteum

Once the subcutaneous tissue is separated from the periosteum by blunt and sharp dissection, a horizontal incision is made in the periosteum inferior to the orbital rim (Figure 3–7:7). A line parallel to the orbital rim and approximately 3 to 4 mm inferior to it is selected. Location of the incision at this level greatly facilitates reapproximation of the cut periosteal edges at the end of the procedure. Also, transection of the orbital septum at its union with the inferior orbital rim is thereby avoided. However, the surgeon should avoid dissecting too far inferiorly and damaging the infraorbital nerve (about 10 mm below the rim). The periosteum should be scraped back over the rim with periosteal elevators, which can then easily strip up the periosteum of the orbital floor in one sheet (Figure 3–7:8). The elevation should continue posteriorly in the floor until the anterior extent of the fracture is met. Then the periosteal elevator should be used to define the extent of the fracture. Care should be taken to elevate the periosteum for the entire medial, lateral, and posterior extent of the fracture. Occasionally this elevation necessitates a far posterior dissection, but its completion is necessary for adequate repair. *Care should be exercised that the globe and the central retinal artery are not inadvertently compressed.*

In delineating the extent of a fracture or of incarcerated tissue, the infraorbital groove or canal is often mistaken for a fracture line and the infraorbital nerve confused with incarcerated tissue. The infraorbital nerve is a terminal branch of the second division of the trigeminal nerve. It enters the orbit through the inferior orbital fissure and traverses the infraorbital canal to reach the face via the infraorbital foramen. Within the infraorbital canal the middle superior and anterior superior dental nerves arise and pass inferiorly to the alveolar arch. The infraorbital groove lies in the floor of the orbit, beginning at about the middle of the inferior orbital fissure, and runs almost straight anteriorly. In its most anterior extent, the groove has a variably formed thin roof of bone; this enclosed portion of the groove is called the infraorbital canal. In some instances the infraorbital canal may be an open groove for its entire extent. It then resembles a fracture line with incarcerated tissue—even more so than normally. Care should be taken not to extract the infraorbital nerves and vessels from such a groove in the mistaken notion that they represent incarcerated orbital tissue. On the other hand, fractures do occasionally occur within the infraorbital groove and should be visible in the preoperative x-rays.

e. *Extrication of Incarcerated Tissue*

Once the limits of the fractures are carefully defined, all incarcerated tissue should be removed. This can be accomplished through a variety of manipulations. With malleable ribbon retractors *gently* holding the orbital tissue superiorly (Figure 3–7:9), periosteal elevators may be used to reach into the bony defect and engage the soft tissues and pull them superiorly out of the fracture site. *Excessive retraction of intraorbital contents jeopardizes the integrity of the central retinal vein and artery.* Gentle traction on the previously placed transconjunctival suture under the inferior rectus muscle may aid in the process of tissue extraction, although care should be taken not to rip the suture through the inferior rectus muscle. *The forced-duction test should be repeated to check for free motility of the globe.*

Occasionally a trapdoor effect has been produced by the fracture, and soft orbital tissue can be withdrawn only by first depressing the plate of bone to relieve the trapping. Fragments of bone should be removed and, if small, discarded. If one or more large plates of bone are free-floating, they should be saved and used to bridge the bony defect. Once the trapped tissue has been removed, the antrum should be suctioned to remove old and fresh blood, loose bone chips, and the like.

f. Caldwell-Luc Approach

Should removal of all incarcerated tissues via the superior vantage point be impossible, an inferior transoral approach to the antrum via a Caldwell-Luc technique should be employed.[9] Because this technique is unfamiliar to most ophthalmic surgeons, the use of a team approach including an otolaryngologist is recommended.

Local anesthesia may be utilized for the Caldwell-Luc operation if necessary, but general anesthesia is infinitely more acceptable for most patients who require bone chiseling. If local anesthesia is employed, the nasal mucosa above and below the inferior turbinate is additionally treated with cocaine-soaked cotton pledgets. Lidocaine containing epinephrine is injected deeply under the periosteum of the canine fossa. The surgical assistant then elevates the upper lip maximally, and an incision through the gingivolabial fold and down to bone is made between the canine and second molar teeth. Using periosteal elevators, the surgeon then strips all the soft tissues off the maxilla (anterior wall of the maxillary antrum) to the level of the infraorbital foramen. Care should be exercised so that the infraorbital nerve and vessels are not injured.

An opening is then made into the antrum with a hammer and a 5-mm chisel. (Occasionally, this procedure will be unnecessary, as the anterior wall of the antrum will be found to be comminuted.) The anterior wall should be chiseled out in as large a single piece as possible. This bone fragment closely conforms in contour and thickness to the normal orbital floor, and it is highly useful for subsequent bridging of the fracture site in the orbit (see below).

Using rongeurs and bone punches, the surgeon then makes an opening into the antrum at least large enough to accommodate a forefinger. It is sometimes impossible to avoid traumatizing some of the alveolar nerves in this process. Blood clots and comminuted bone fragments are removed. The larger bony fragments can then be pulled downward, and the trapped orbital tissues can simultaneously be pushed up (by any of the techniques previously mentioned). Any hinged flap of orbital floor bone should then be elevated back into position.

Next, a large nasoantral window is made by inserting a Kelly clamp relatively far posteriorly under the inferior turbinate; the clamp is then simply pushed laterally through the thin medial wall of the antrum. The opening produced in this fashion is enlarged by spreading and rotating the jaws of the clamp.

In making the nasoantral window, trauma to the ostium of the nasolacrimal duct is rarely produced. Such trauma can be avoided by recalling that this ostium is most commonly located 3 to 4 cm posterior to the nostril (one fourth the way back in the inferior meatus of the nose) and just below the attached border of the inferior turbinate, i.e., in the anterior and superior aspect of the lateral wall of the inferior meatus. Thus, the Kelly clamp should be kept as far inferior as possible when pushing it from the nose into the antrum. The ideal nasoantral window will thus be inferior and posterior to the ostium of the nasolacrimal canal.

A long, antibiotic-soaked gauze strip packing the antrum keeps the elevated orbital floor fragments in their normal position. *Excessive packing should be avoided* because a hypertropia can result, pressure can be transmitted to the optic nerve and its blood vessels, and pressure can be acutely and severely elevated within the globe itself.

The antral packing is next drawn into the inferior meatus of the nose. At this time, bone spicules in the nasoantral window should be smoothed out lest they subsequently catch the gauze packing and interfere with its removal through the nostril. Elimination of the spicules can be accomplished by bone punches or by vigorously pulling the packing back and forth through the nasoantral opening in a sawing fashion. The packing is left extending into the inferior meatus far enough to be visible in the nostril. The gingival incision is closed with absorbable sutures. The packing is removed through the nostril with the patient under mild sedation on approximately the tenth postoperative day. An alternative, though less desirable, technique of packing eliminates the nasal antrostomy. The antral packing is simply carried out through the gingivolabial incision, from which it is subsequently removed.

Some surgeons prefer to eliminate the skin incision completely and attempt to reduce the fracture exclusively via the Caldwell-Luc approach.[9] In rare instances, such as patients with coincident lid injuries, this operation may be indicated. In most cases, however, it is not justified, since it is difficult to determine if all tissue has been freed of its incarceration. It is also more difficult to assess over- or underpacking of the antrum with the Caldwell-Luc approach than when the orbital floor is under direct visualization from above.

g. Sealing the Fracture

Whenever possible, local bone plates should be kept in situ to bridge the fracture. Occasionally, the bone has been comminuted to the point that no useable material remains. On the other hand, blow-out fractures of the orbit are frequently hinged on one side, and the plate of bone can be elevated into normal position. This can be accomplished through the use, for example, of blunt muscle hooks or skin hooks from above (occasionally, considerable force is required); a Caldwell-Luc approach can be used but is not usually necessary.

If sufficient bone is not present locally for restoration of the orbital floor, a variety of other materials should be used. A convenient material for this purpose is Supramid in sheet form (0.3-mm thick). Sheets of Supramid can be sterilized by autoclaving or gas exposure. They are stiff enough to prevent herniation into the antrum, thin enough to avoid an induced hypertropia, and soft enough to be cut with scissors at the operating table. They are also virtually inert and do not adhere to tissues; if necessary, they can be easily removed postoperatively.

The Supramid sheet should be cut in the shape of a lancet or an isosceles triangle with rounded corners. It is then placed between the periosteum and the bone of the orbital floor, with its apex pointed posteriorly (Figure 3–7:10). It should be large enough to extend at least 3 mm beyond all fractured bone but small enough that it does not encroach on the periosteum of the inferior orbital rim anteriorly, on the lacrimal fossa anteromedially, or on the contents of the inferior orbital fissure posteriorly. Occasionally, a notch cut in the posterior apex of the Supramid sheet can accommodate the structures of the inferior orbital fissure. Under most circumstances, the Supramid sheet does not have to be sutured in position. However, if the fracture is extensive and downward migration of the Supramid appears inevitable, suturing the sheet to bone or periosteum can easily be accomplished. Similarly, large, unstable bone fragments should be wired into position during this stage of the operation. Anterior migration can be prevented in some cases by cutting a hinge in the anterior border of the implant.

A large variety of living as well as preserved human tissues have been used for restitution of the orbital floor. An equally large variety of alloplastics other than Supramid have also been employed, including methyl methacrylate, polyethylene, silicone, and Teflon. Rapidly polymerizing as well as preformed plastics are now commercially available.

Bone and cartilage grafts are the most commonly employed human derivatives. If bone from the canine fossa is not available, the iliac crest is a convenient source of human bone for this purpose, but in preparing this tissue, care should be taken to make the plate of bone quite thin (no thicker than 3 mm). A severe hypertropia can result if the material used to bridge the fracture is too thick. The pain and discomfort from iliac bone surgery usually outlast the pain and discomfort emanating from facial surgery.

h. Closure

The periosteum should be closed with interrupted absorbable sutures (Figure 3–7:11).

It is rarely necessary to place sutures in the orbicularis muscle or other subcutaneous tissue, since the blunt muscle-splitting dissection (see Figure 3–7:6) promotes spontaneous reapproximation.

The skin can be closed by any acceptable suture technique (Figure 3–7:12). A mild pressure dressing should be applied to minimize orbital and lid swelling, but the pressure should not be so intense that occlusion of the central retinal artery is likely.

i. Postoperative Care and Clinical Course

Vision should be checked every four to six hours during the first day to be certain that hematoma formation has not resulted in compression of the central retinal artery. If antral packing has been performed, intraocular pressure should be measured to be certain that overpacking has not compressed the globe.

Most patients are treated for the first one or two postoperative days with cold compresses or ice packs to minimize lid and orbital edema. Subsequently, warm compresses are applied to enhance local circulation and to hasten resorption of interstitial fluids.

A broad-spectrum antibiotic is usually administered systemically for seven to ten days, since direct contamination of intraorbital tissues with antral contents is unavoidable. An orally administered decongestant such as pseudoephedrine is routinely used in an effort to shrink the sinus mucosa and promote adequate sinus drainage.

Postoperative limitation of ocular motility is commonplace, and in the immediate postoperative period it should not be construed as the result of an inadequate operation. Frequently, weeks and sometimes months pass before full ocular motility is required. Marked orbital and lid swelling, however, are uncommon; if persistent or exaggerated, these symptoms should suggest the presence of postoperative cellulitis, abscess, osteomyelitis, or sinusitis.

j. Intraoperative Complications of Surgery

Inability to Extricate All Incarcerated Tissue. Should soft-tissue incarceration in the fracture site remain after repeated attempts at removal from the superior approach, the surgeon has no recourse but to perform an antrostomy in the Caldwell-Luc fashion. Combined manipulations from above and below will relieve the entrapment in almost all circumstances.

Avulsion of the Inferior Rectus or Inferior Oblique Muscle. Should the conjoint fascial investment of the inferior rectus muscle and the inferior oblique muscle (Lockwood's ligament) be incarcerated in the fracture site, vigorous traction from above can result in avulsion or transection of either one or both of these muscles. Unnecessary manipulation of the muscle tissue should be avoided.

Mistaken Identification of the Infraorbital Nerve, Vessel, or Groove.
Should the infraorbital nerve, vessel, or groove be mistaken for a fracture
with incarcerated tissue, extensive and irreparable trauma can result from
an attempt to manipulate any of these structures. Needless to say,
adequate knowledge of the normal anatomy of the orbital floor is essential
to successful surgery.

Excessive Pressure on the Globe. Throughout the exposure of the
orbital floor, the orbital contents must be retracted superiorly. In doing
so, it is all too easy to exert unnecessary pressure on the globe itself,
leading to central retinal artery occlusion. Exquisite concern for this
extraordinarily severe complication should be maintained throughout the
operation.

k. Postoperative Complications

Bacterial Contamination. Exposure of the intraorbital contents to the
maxillary sinus causes immediate bacterial contamination. In the vast
majority of cases, no untoward sequelae occur. However, postoperative
cellulitis should be suspected and should be adequately cultured and
treated if postoperative edema, chemosis, limitation of gaze, or exophthalmos persists or worsens.

Persistent Limitation in Vertical Gaze. Limitation in vertical gaze is
commonplace immediately after operation, and it may persist in some
degree for weeks or possibly even for a month or two. Therefore, re-
exploration of the orbital floor during the immediate postoperative course
is almost never justified unless definite limitation of the forced ductions
occurs after initial improvement. Should symptomatic gaze limitation
remain permanently, repair via surgery on the extraocular muscles themselves should be attempted after six to nine months have elapsed since
the initial surgery. Minor deviations can sometimes be treated with
spectacle prisms. Recession of the inferior and superior rectus muscles
has been reported to increase the field of single vision in patients with
orbital floor fractures.[10]

Persistent Exophthalmos. Excessive graft material in the fracture site
will invariably produce hypertropia and some degree of exophthalmos.
These complications should be prevented; otherwise, re-exploration of the
orbital floor with removal of the extra material will be necessary.

Enophthalmos. Enophthalmos may be the result of failure to extract
all incarcerated orbital tissue, an incompletely bridged fracture (with
subsequent reincarceration of orbital fat), or traumatic fat atrophy. If an
antrostomy has been performed, enophthalmos can result from underpacking of the sinus.

Extrusion of the Alloplastic Sheet. The sheet of artificial material
used to bridge the fracture site may migrate anteriorly and present as a

tender mass in the lower lid. This complication can be largely avoided at the time of initial surgery by carefully reapproximating the periosteum of the inferior orbital rim or by suturing the implant to the adjacent bone. Should significant intraorbital infection occur, however, even such assiduous care may not prevent extrusion of the sheet. The only recourse then is to remove the sheet through a lower lid incision and provide whatever drainage is necessary. Fortunately, this complication is rather uncommon.

Lower Lid Ectropion. Ectropion of the lower lid may result from a number of causes. If, in repairing the periosteal incision at the inferior rim, traction is placed on the inferior orbital septum, postoperative ectropion can result. Furthermore, a cutaneous incision at the level of the inferior orbital rim may, on occasion, scar down to the underlying periosteal incision and contribute to formation of a lower lid ectropion. Should any postoperative lid infection occur, the ectropion will be exacerbated by the resulting scar formation.

Postoperative Lid Edema. Several mechanisms may be responsible for postoperative edema of the lid. Localized pockets of interstitial fluid may persist if the orbicularis muscle is reapproximated with large sutures; usually, such suturing is not required. In addition, it appears that cutaneous and orbicularis incisions that run too horizontally can interrupt lymphatic drainage. The normal lymphatic drainage from the lateral part of the lower lid is via vessels that run inferolaterally to the superficial parotid lymph nodes and superficial cervical lymph nodes. Therefore, with both the lower lid fold incision and the inferior orbital rim incision, it appears wise to angle the lateral extent of the incision somewhat inferiorly in an attempt to minimize transection of the draining lymphatics. Otherwise, postoperative lid edema may persist for months.

Dacryocystitis. Postoperative dacryocystitis is sometimes unavoidable, especially when the lacrimal bone or nasolacrimal duct is fractured by the initial trauma (Figure 3–8). However, care in reflecting the anteromedial periosteum of the orbital floor can help prevent damage to an otherwise intact lacrimal sac. Insertion of bone grafts or alloplastics between the periosteum and the bony floor of the orbit should be accomplished without impinging on the lacrimal fossa. If postoperative dacryocystitis occurs despite such careful manipulations, it is treated with antibiotics, irrigations, probings, and, if necessary, dacryocystorhinostomy.

Blindness and Acute Elevation of Intraocular Pressure. Within several hours after surgery to repair a blow-out fracture, vision may be severely reduced, even to the point of no light perception. Intraoperative trauma to the optic nerve (from periosteal elevators, retractors, the subperiosteal implant, or overpacking of the antrum) may cause immediate loss of vision. Postoperative orbital hemorrhage (Figure 3–9) associated with acute, severe pain and progressive loss of vision requires immediate

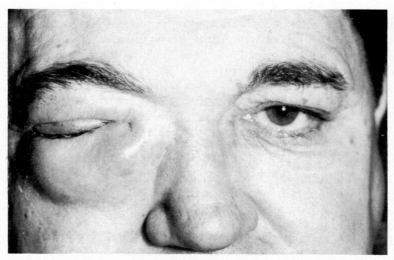

Figure 3–8. Dacryocystitis. This condition can be a late complication of orbital blow-out fracture, maxillary fracture, or severance of lacrimal duct.

orbital decompression by removal of the subperiosteal implant, drainage of any hematoma, and removal of antral packing.[11] Restoration of vision may occur if immediate surgery is undertaken.

Overpacking of the antrum (with such material as gauze or balloons) may seriously elevate intraocular pressure. Frequent postoperative moni-

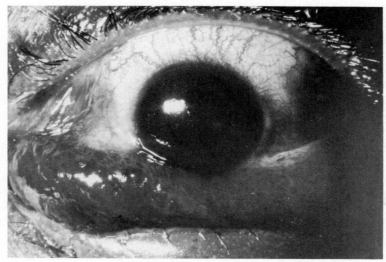

Figure 3–9. Orbital hemorrhage with proptosis and large subconjunctival hematoma preventing lid closure, subsequent to repair of orbital floor fracture.

toring of pupillary reactivity, visual acuity, intraocular pressure, and fundus appearance is mandatory, for occlusion of the central retinal artery has been reported as a complication after repair of a blow-out fracture.[12]

3.3 MEDIAL WALL AND SUPERIOR WALL ORBITAL FRACTURES

a. Medial Wall Fractures

Fractures of the medial wall of the orbit are not infrequently observed in combination with fractures of the orbital floor,[13, 14] but they may also be observed as isolated complications of blunt orbital trauma (Fig. 3–10). In either case, suspicion of medial wall involvement is raised when there is orbital or lid emphysema, epistaxis, limitation of abduction, or an acquired retraction syndrome (the last two physical signs are due to entrapment of the medial rectus muscle). Both cutaneous and conjunctival incisions can be used in approaching the site of entrapment.[14, 15]

b. Superior Wall Fractures

Although rare, fractures of the superior wall are potentially dangerous because of the possibility of intracranial hemorrhage or infection. In addition, injury to the levator palpebrae superioris and superior rectus muscles or their nerve supplies can induce ptosis and weakness of

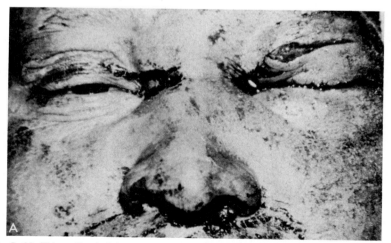

Figure 3–10. This patient's left eye was struck with the full force of a high-pressure fire hose. (A) When first seen after the injury, lid contours were flat, and no globe was present in the orbit.

Illustration continued on following page

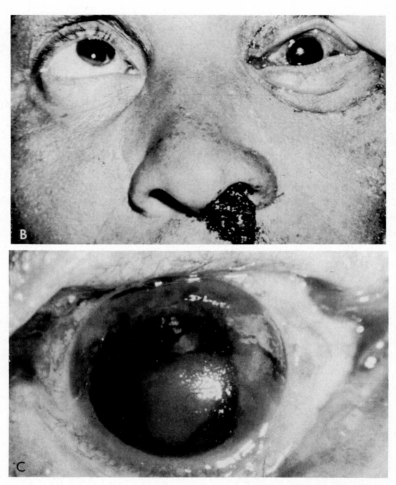

Figure 3–10. *Continued.* (B) The force of the water had blasted the globe into the ethmoid sinus, from which it was retrieved by manipulation through the nose combined with traction from the palpebral fissure. (C) The globe on restoration to its proper position. There is fibrin in the anterior chamber. (Photographs published through the courtesy of James B. Wise. M.D.)

supraduction. Injuries to the lacrimal gland, optic nerve, and intracranial structures may also occur.[16, 17]

3.4 TRIMALAR FRACTURES

Fractures arising from blunt trauma to the zygomatic bone may cause dislocation of this bone, thereby creating multiple orbital fractures. Such zygomatic bone fractures are commonly called *tripod* or *trimalar* fractures[18] because of the characteristic sites of bony separation: the lateral orbital rim, the infraorbital rim, and the zygomatic arch. Since a fracture in the infraorbital rim usually extends posteriorly into the floor of the orbit, physical signs similar to those indicating isolated blow-out fractures of the floor may be observed.

The typical line of a complete, dislocating fracture of the zygomatic bone involves the lateral orbital rim at or near the zygomaticofrontal suture line. From this rim, the fracture line continues posteriorly and inferiorly along the lateral orbital wall to reach the infraorbital fissure, then continues anteriorly in the floor of the orbit to reach the infraorbital rim near the infraorbital canal. From this point, it runs inferiorly and laterally along or near the zygomaticomaxillary suture line. Often, the zygomatic arch is also fractured.[18]

The indications for the surgical repair of these injuries are inability to open the mouth (trismus) and unacceptable facial asymmetry. Permanent reduction of these fractures usually necessitates wiring of the orbital margin.

References

1. Anderson RL, Panje WR, Gross CE: Optic nerve blindness following blunt forehead trauma. Ophthalmology 89:445–455, 1982.
2. Gilbard SM, Mafee MF, Lagouros PA, Langer BG: The prognostic significance of computed tomography of orbital blowout fractures. (In press.)
3. Crikelair GF, Rein JM, Potter GD, Cosman B: A critical look at the blowout fracture. Plast Reconstr Surg 49:374–379, 1972.
4. Emery JM, Craig JA: A review of techniques of blow-out fracture surgery. Surv Ophthalmol, in press.
5. Emery JM, von Noorden GK, Schlernitzauer DA: Orbital floor fractures: long-term follow-up of cases with and without surgical repair. Trans Am Acad Ophthalmol Otolaryngol 75:802–812, 1971.
6. Emery JM, von Noorden GK, Schlernitzauer DA: Management of orbital floor fractures. Am J Ophthalmol 74:299–306, 1972.
7. Putterman AM, Stevens T, Urist-MJ: Nonsurgical management of blow-out fractures of the orbital floor. Am J Ophthalmol 77:232–239, 1974.
8. Atlee WE Jr: Talc and cornstarch emboli in eyes of drug abusers. JAMA 219:49–51, 1972.
9. Walter WL: Early surgical repair of blowout fracture of the orbital floor by using the transantral approach. South Med J 65:1229–1243, 1972.
10. Kushner BJ: Paresis and restriction of the inferior rectus muscle after orbital floor fracture. Am J Ophthalmol 94:81–86, 1982.
11. Nicholson DH, Guzak SV Jr: Visual loss complicating repair of orbital floor fractures. Arch Ophthalmol 86:369–375, 1971.
12. Emery JM, Huff JD, and Justice J Jr: Central retinal artery occlusion after blow-out fracture repair. Am J Ophthalmol 78:538–540, 1974.
13. Dodick JM, Galin MA, Littleton JT, Sod LM: Concomitant medial wall fracture and blowout fracture of the orbit. Arch Ophthalmol 85:273–276, 1971.
14. Rumelt MB, Ernest JT: Isolated blowout fracture of medial orbital wall with medial rectus muscle entrapment. Am J Ophthalmol 73:451–453, 1972.
15. Schonder AA, Salz JJ, Magnus WW, Castner DV Jr: A conjunctival approach to repair of fracture of medial wall of orbit: case report. Ann Ophthalmol 4:297–308, 1972.
16. Smith RR, Blount RL: Blowout fracture of the orbital roof with pulsating exophthalmos, blepharoptosis and superior gaze paresis. Am J Ophthalmol 71:1052–1054, 1971.
17. McLachlan DL, Flanagan JC, Shannon GM: Complications of orbital roof fractures. Ophthalmology 89:1274–1278, 1982.
18. Hotte HHA: Orbital Fractures. Springfield, Ill, Charles C Thomas Co, 1970.

Intraocular and Intraorbital Foreign Bodies

Whenever periorbital or ocular tissues are lacerated or punctured, the physician must rule out the presence of a retained intraorbital or intraocular foreign body (Table 4–1). Medicolegal considerations as well as economic realities have resulted in added impetus for the development of accurate and efficient means of diagnosing and localizing intraocular and intraorbital foreign bodies.

Optimal clinical management depends largely on the following factors: (1) accurate localization of the foreign body; (2) knowledge of its composition, shape, and size; (3) delineation of the extent of the ocular

Table 4–1. EVALUATION OF INTRAOCULAR FOREIGN BODIES

1. Careful history.
2. Physical examination.
3. Drawing of location of foreign body.
4. CT scan if foreign body suspected but not visualized.
5. Bone-free x-rays to distinguish intraocular from soft tissue foreign bodies in the anterior segment.
6. Determination or confirmation of magnetic characteristics.
7. Culture of the object from which the foreign body came.
8. Intravenous antibiotics.
9. Preparation for surgery.

Table 4–2. QUESTIONS RELATED TO POSSIBLE INTRAOCULAR FOREIGN BODY

Circumstances of the injury
1. How did the injury occur?
2. Was it self-inflicted?
3. Was it accidental or intentional?
4. Did it occur in connection with the patient's work?
5. Was the patient wearing safety glasses or other protective devices?
6. Was the patient inebriated?

Chronology of events
1. What was the exact time of injury?
2. What activities occurred after injury, e.g., bending, stooping, or lifting heavy objects?
3. When did the patient last take anything by mouth; i.e., when can he safely undergo anesthesia, if necessary?

Previous therapy
1. Was the patient seen or treated by other professional personnel? What are their names, and how can they be contacted?
2. If ocular or other therapy was instituted, what was its nature?
3. Has the patient had tetanus immunization? If so, when? Is the patient allergic to tetanus antitoxin? (See Table 8–2)

Pretraumatic condition
1. Prior to injury, did the involved eye have normal vision or pre-existent disease? Is the uninjured eye normal?

Foreign-body involvement
1. Was a foreign body or missile involved? If so
   a. Is its composition known?
   b. If it is metal, what type? *Is it magnetic?*
   c. If a missile originated from the use of tools, what objects were involved: e.g., iron hammer on steel chisel on concrete; steel axe on wood containing nails; wood hammer on steel screwdriver on brass rod?
2. Were spectacles worn? Were they safety glasses? Were they struck by the foreign body? Are the lenses and frames intact?
3. Could there be intracranial extension of the injury?

or orbital trauma; (4) the appropriate decision regarding whether to remove the foreign body or leave it in place; and (5) technical competence in the actual removal of the foreign body and the management of any intraoperative complications that may develop.[1, 2]

In eliciting the patient's history, precise and minute details of the injury should be obtained. In particular, the questions listed in Table 4–2 should be among those answered.

4.1 DIAGNOSIS

a. Common Sites

Sites of foreign bodies within the eye and beneath the lids are shown in Figure 4–1. Intraocular foreign bodies are retained in the following sites:

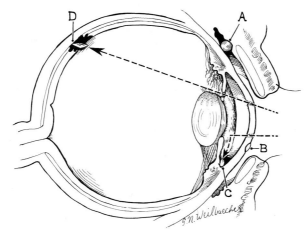

Figure 4–1. Common sites of foreign bodies. (A) Particles such as BB pellets and even contact lenses may be retained in the conjunctival fornix of the upper lid. (B) Corneal foreign bodies are usually found within the lid fissure. (C) Small, sharp particles such as glass fragments may pass through the cornea and sink into the angle of the anterior chamber inferiorly. (D) Metallic missiles may pass through the cornea, iris, and lens and lodge in the posterior wall of the eye or remain within the vitreous cavity. Less frequently, they pass entirely through the eye and remain within the orbit.

15 per cent in the anterior chamber; 8 per cent in the lens; 70 per cent in the posterior segment; and 7 per cent in the orbit (double perforation).[3] Detection of a single foreign body in any one of these sites can provide the examiner with a false sense of security because multiple foreign bodies are not uncommon. This is especially true after a barrage of missiles from explosions, shotgun blasts, and the like (Figure 4–2).

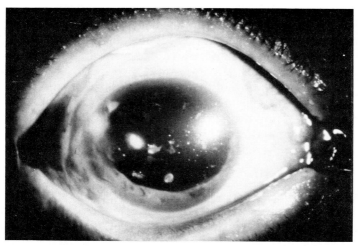

Figure 4–2. Intracorneal rocks after a blasting injury. This patient was injured when a blasting cap, which was being embedded in the earth, exploded prematurely. Several rocks were found within each cornea and lens. This eye has undergone a pars plana lensectomy and vitrectomy to remove retained debris.

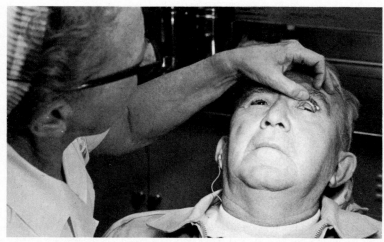

Figure 4–3. Simple eversion of the upper lid demonstrated with the patient in a comfortable sitting position.

Eversion of the upper lid (Figures 4–3, 4–4, and 4–5) is extremely important in the routine search for small missiles that have struck the eye. Double eversion of the upper lid (see Figure 4–5) is sometimes required for visualization of a foreign body in the depths of the superior conjunctival cul-de-sac. Foreign bodies may also be concealed in the inferior fornix or even in the lacrimal sac.[4] Fragments of glass or transparent plastic are often highly elusive. They may be obscured by mucus or by a fold of conjunctiva, or fragments may be hidden beneath the plica semilunaris.

A very common etiology of intraocular foreign bodies is a "metal on metal" injury. Often, the patient has been beating (or watching someone else beat) a piece of metal with a metal hammer when the injury occurs. The foreign body is often a piece of the hammer, which has become weakened after years of use. In this case the hammer should be inspected, and if a chip is missing, the hammer should be cultured and tested to see if it is magnetic. While the foreign body is often sterilized by the heat energy used in creating it, this should never be assumed, and the patient should receive prophylactic antibiotics.

b. Direct Visualization

Various techniques are available for determining the presence and location of intraorbital and intraocular foreign bodies. However, it cannot be overemphasized that *direct visualization of the object by the physician far surpasses any other means of foreign-body detection.*

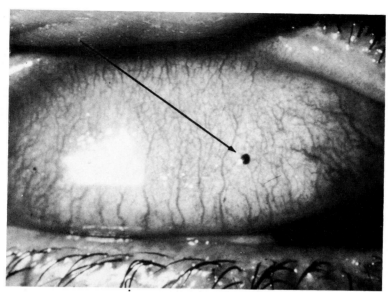

Figure 4–4. A common location for air-borne dust particles is the tarsal conjunctiva (arrow). Vertical "scratch marks" on the cornea are demonstrated with fluorescein staining and suggest the tarsal location of the foreign body. For removal of a foreign body on the tarsal conjunctiva with a cotton-tipped applicator, no anesthetic solution is required, and eye patching is unnecessary in most cases.

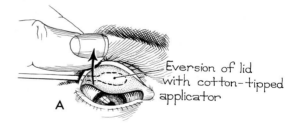

Eversion of lid with cotton-tipped applicator

A

Figure 4–5. Techniques of single and double eversion of the upper lid.

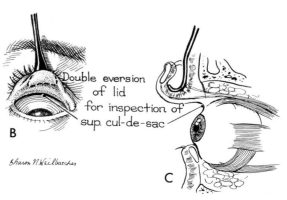

Double eversion of lid for inspection of sup. cul-de-sac

B

Sharon N.Weilbacher

C

Small foreign bodies in the anterior segment of the eye can be difficult to identify even with a slit lamp (Figure 4–6). They can be hidden within iris crypts or surrounded by blood. Especially when rusty, they can also be confused with an iris nevus or an avulsed section of iris sphincter or pigment epithelium. A tiny iris perforation made by a foreign body may be small enough to be invisible with *direct* illumination (Figure 4–7). Iris *transillumination* by directing a light through the pupil can produce a red

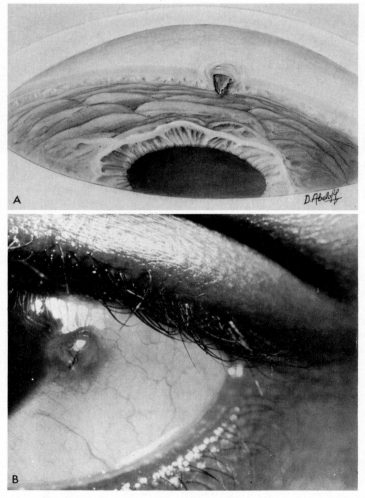

Figure 4–6. Retained paralimbal foreign body. (A) A lodged chip of brick, penetrating obliquely through the trabecular meshwork into the anterior chamber. (B) The foreign body, reportedly retained for several years, had produced a paralimbal bleb with chronic external drainage of aqueous. (This case was reported by Morse PH: Paralimbal foreign body with filtering effect. Am J Ophthalmol 66:92–95, 1968.)

fundus reflex through the iris defect if the lens and vitreous are not opaque. Direct visualization of the anterior chamber angle with a gonioprism is sometimes useful in detecting an otherwise hidden foreign body. However, gonioscopy can produce a leak of aqueous through a recently penetrated cornea. A clue to the presence and location of such a foreign body is focal bedewing, or *epithelial edema of the peripheral cornea,* but this may not develop for months after injury.

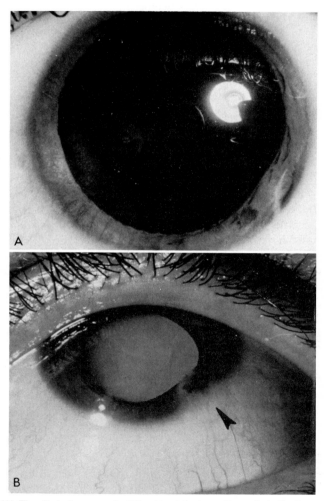

Figure 4–7. (A) Tiny limbal scar and slitlike iris defect are the only indications of the site of entry of a metallic chip that passed through the lens and zonule and came to rest within the vitreous. (B) Traumatic cataract resulting from perforating injury. Note limbal injury site (arrow). The case illustrated here resulted from perforation of the eye by a sharp foreign body that was withdrawn. The anterior chamber has re-formed. The significance of the injury remained unrecognized until the eventual development of a cataract. These two figures exemplify the diversity of consequences that can result from similar injuries at almost identical sites.

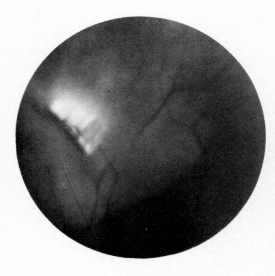

Figure 4–8. Intravitreal foreign body. While pounding on a metal bolt with a metal hammer, this patient felt a foreign body sensation but suffered no decrease in acuity. After dilatation of the pupil, the examiner found this metallic foreign body within the vitreous body.

Should the foreign body lie in the vitreous or on the retina, *no single form of examination is more effective than ophthalmoscopy* (Figure 4–8). Particularly with indirect ophthalmoscopy, the surgeon can most precisely determine the proper therapeutic course of action. In many cases, the exact position and nature of the foreign body can be determined; a posterior wound of exit can be seen (with or without retinal incarceration); trauma to the disc and macula can be assessed; ricochet wounds in the retina and concomitant vitreous and retinal hemorrhage or detachment can be documented. Because these factors are critically important, maximum pupillary dilatation and indirect ophthalmoscopy should be performed (after slit-lamp examination) when a foreign body posterior to the iris is suspected. Since traumatic lenticular perforations can lead to rapid onset of a cataract (sometimes within minutes or hours) and since hemorrhage into the vitreous may disperse and cloud the media with equal rapidity, *the first examiner may be the only one able to examine the posterior portion of the eye.* Such examination must never be delayed and should be given urgent priority. A few moments should be taken to make a drawing of the location of any intravitreal or retinal foreign bodies, as they often become hard to locate under the microscope during the operation.

Once opacification of the ocular media occurs, the therapeutic decision-making becomes much more difficult. Precise localization of the foreign body, possible retinal detachment, and possible choroidal hemorrhage and detachment are among the important diagnoses that become difficult to make without visualization.

Some foreign bodies remain "silent" and undetectable by routine biomicroscopy and ophthalmoscopy. A variety of clues provide evidence that the eye harbors such objects: focal bedewing; a biomicroscopically visible corneal, lenticular, or vitreous tract; angle trauma with peripheral anterior synechias or angle recession; iridotomy or iridodialysis; heterochromia; anisocoria or pupillary irregularity; sector zonulolysis; and persistent uveitis or hypopyon.

c. Indirect Demonstration

Should visualization of the foreign body be impossible, the radiologic techniques discussed in Chapter 6 are the next recourse. Briefly, plain orbital x-rays, bone-free films, and computerized tomograms are the most useful techniques in this regard. The availability of these modalities has virtually eliminated the need for the older and less accurate triangulation localization techniques of past years.

Modern A-scan and B-scan ultrasonography has also improved the ophthalmologist's ability to detect and localize foreign bodies. While ultrasonography can probably be as accurate as x-ray techniques in experienced hands, such expertise is not as readily available as high-quality radiologic assistance.

Precise localizations can often be obtained with *electronic foreign body locators.*[5] Some of these instruments can also determine whether or not a foreign body is magnetic. Indeed, the knowledge that a foreign body is or is not magnetic is almost essential in the planning of the removal procedure. Iron and ordinary carbon steel are most easily detected by foreign-body locators such as the Berman apparatus (Figure 4–9). The detecting range for an iron-containing object is about ten times the diameter of the foreign body; i.e., a 1-mm iron particle can be detected at about 10 mm. Alloy and stainless steel produce a poorer response by this instrument. Pure nickel is magnetic and is thus easily detected, but coin nickel is nonmagnetic and is less easily located. Other nonmagnetic metals, including brass, copper, lead, and aluminum, induce a much weaker response than does iron or steel; i.e., nonmagnetic foreign bodies may be detectable only within one to two times their own diameter. Thus, in practical terms, the size of a nonmagnetic foreign body within the eye must be greater than 3 mm in order for it to be detected by the Berman locator. The sensitivity of the Berman locator to nonmagnetic metals is directly proportional to the electrical conductivity of the metal; e.g., silver > copper > aluminum > brass > lead, and so forth.

In summary, the response evoked from a metal-detecting device is not only related to the size of the metallic fragment but also depends on magnetic properties of the metal or its conductive properties or both. Locators are most valuable for precise detection of a foreign body embedded posteriorly in the wall of the eye when direct trans-scleral cutdown

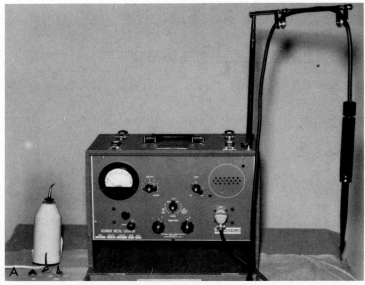

Figure 4–9. (A) The Berman metal locator (right) and a small electromagnet with assorted tips (left). Both instruments have sterile covers for use in the operating room. Because foreign bodies within the vitreous can be shifted at the time of surgical manipulation of the eye, the use of a locator at the time of operation is often of major importance in deciding on the best location for the scleral incision.

Illustration continued on opposite page

and extraction are planned. They are similarly useful at the time of surgery for differentiating an intraocular from an extraocular location if the x-rays were not useful in this regard.[6]

4.2 PROGNOSIS AND COMPLICATIONS

a. Prognosis

Once an intraocular location of a foreign body has been established, the prognosis is always guarded; useful vision and the globe itself can be lost in a variety of ways. The initial determination must be whether or not enucleation is justified (see Chapter 8). As in the case of corneal and scleral lacerations without foreign bodies, immediate enucleation is rarely advisable. Neither the patient's well-being nor the health of the other eye is jeopardized by delaying enucleation for several days. Remarkable recovery may reward perseverance. The persistence of good light projection is a frequent indication for delaying enucleation. However, as in all cases of perforating injury, consideration for the potential development of sympathetic ophthalmia is an absolute requirement (see Chapter 8).

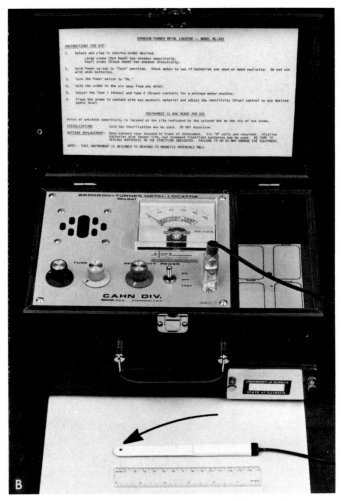

Figure 4–9. *(Continued).* (B) The Bronson-Turner metal locator. Note probe (arrow).

Careful biomicroscopic evaluation of the nonpenetrated eye should be part of the daily examination ritual to determine if there are early signs of inflammation. Any definitive therapy should take into account the possibility of enucleating the injured eye within the first five to ten days of the traumatic episode in an effort to forestall the development of sympathetic ophthalmia. If good visual acuity remains and the perforation can be surgically repaired without significant damage to the eye, attempts to retain the injured eye are surely justified. In making the decision whether or not to enucleate the injured eye, the perforating effects of the trauma must be assessed in conjunction with the blunt contusive effects,

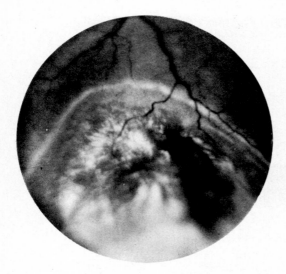

Figure 4–10. Postoperative appearance of patient in Figure 4–8. Following removal of the foreign body, a retinal hole that matched the shape of the metallic fragment was discovered, implying that the piece had bounced off the retinal surface. Because there was a small retinal detachment surrounding the hole, a radial scleral sponge was placed over the hole. The postoperative visual acuity was 20/15.

the immediate chemical effects, and the immediate inflammatory effects. In addition, an informed judgment as to the probable consequences of subsequent chemical, inflammatory, and reparative processes must be included in the overall appraisal of the clinical situation.

At the time of initial surgical repair of the wound of entry, apparently hopeless situations characterized by gaping wounds, avulsed tissue, prolapsed intraocular contents, and extensive hemorrhage can occasionally be converted into much more favorable circumstances by meticulous surgical restoration. If accurate light projection is lost during the first or second post-traumatic week, enucleation is probably in the best interest of the patient. Ultrasound is useful in assessing whether or not the retina is detached. Occasionally, immediate enucleation is justified, as in the case of total disruption of the globe from a bullet's direct hit. All remnants of the globe should be removed.

Since intraocular foreign bodies can cause ricochet wounds in the retina or can produce double perforations, complete retinal evaluation should be performed in salvageable cases so that any retinal break or scleral wound of exit can be treated at the time of closure of the wound of entry or foreign-body extraction (Figure 4–10).

Foreign bodies containing iron or copper (or compounds that can liberate these elements) are particularly dangerous. The clinical syndromes induced by these metals are siderosis and chalcosis, respectively.

b. Complications

Siderosis. Siderosis is a late-occurring syndrome caused by retained foreign bodies of iron or steel. The initial effects are primarily mechanical and contusive rather than chemical. It is uncommon for these intraocular foreign bodies to cause infections, for they often originate from metal striking on metal, and this usually induces enough heat to sterilize them.

Whether siderosis will occur depends largely on the ferrous content of the metal. Various other results are possible, including: no reaction at all, perhaps because of low ferrous content or fibrous encapsulation; no initial reaction, but late inflammation after a shift in the position of an encapsulated foreign body; phthisis bulbi from recurrent inflammation; spontaneous expulsion of the foreign body from the globe; total dissolution of the foreign body without siderosis; and sympathetic ophthalmia, an uncommon but dreaded complication.[3]

In siderosis, ferrous pigmentation causes a rusty coloration of the cornea, iris, or lens. In addition, a series of chronic degenerative changes may lead to cataract, pigmentary degeneration of the retina (with poor night vision and constricted fields), retinal detachment, or open-angle glaucoma (apparently due to iron-containing phagocytes and cell debris blocking the trabecular meshwork).[7] These complications usually occur between two months and two years after the injury but may occur within several days. They are severe enough to warrant major surgical attempts to extract the foreign body as soon as possible after injury (Figure 4–11).

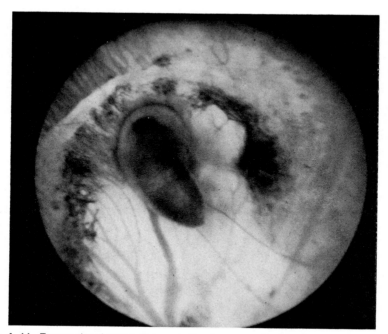

Figure 4–11. Encapsulated metal fragment. For ten years the eye has retained a metallic foreign body that was not detected at the time of original injury. Encapsulation of the metal fragment by a dense fibrous tissue coating has undoubtedly minimized toxic effects of the metal, but early siderosis is now occurring. Whenever possible, metallic foreign bodies should be removed soon after the injury. This eye may eventually be lost as a result of the complication of siderosis bulbi.

Chalcosis. Copper and its common alloys, bronze and brass, may induce chalcosis, a set of chronic degenerative processes in the eye. If the copper content of the foreign body is high, however, a most serious reaction, including hypopyon and localized (sterile) abscesses within the eye, can occur quickly (within several days). This acute chalcosis mimics pyogenic endophthalmitis but has not been positively shown to respond significantly to antibiotics and corticosteroids used in human subjects. An attempt at surgical removal is therefore indicated when this diagnosis is made.

Chalcosis is ordinarily induced by slow diffusion of copper, with preferential deposition of the metal on the basement membranes of the eye. This is in contradistinction to siderosis bulbi, in which the iron is preferentially deposited intracellularly, particularly in epithelial-type cells. A Kayser-Fleischer ring in Descemet's membrane and a sunflower cataract in the anterior capsule of the lens are particularly impressive manifestations of chalcosis, and they resemble those seen in Wilson's hepatolenticular degeneration. Late onset of chalcosis is similar to that of siderosis, but the ocular prognosis is not nearly as poor. Consequently, immediate removal of foreign bodies with a low copper content is not nearly as imperative as it is in cases with retained iron. Indeed, some eyes can retain copper-containing foreign bodies for surprisingly long times without significant loss of vision.[8] Since copper and its alloys are nonmagnetic, the difficulty of removal is an additional justification for a more conservative policy. Some ultimate vision loss due to retained copper-containing foreign bodies is likely, because destruction of retinal neurons and other toxic manifestations often occur, but before attempting surgical removal of a nonmagnetic foreign body the ophthalmologist must always evaluate the possibility of immediate or eventual loss of vision as the direct result of such a hazardous maneuver.

Other Reactions. Other metals typically produce inflammatory reactions somewhat less intense than those from copper and iron. *In decreasing order of ocular reactivity,* they are mercury, aluminum, nickel, zinc, and lead. Except for pure nickel, these metals are nonmagnetic. Other foreign bodies, such as the precious metals, stone, carbon, porcelain, glass, dried building plaster, and various rubbers, are *usually* inert in the eye, although sharp edges can cause mechanical damage. Therefore, an attempt at removal should be performed only if the foreign body is immediately accessible, as in the anterior chamber. Even then, operative intervention for small particles is not necessarily indicated.

c. *Electroretinogram*

The course of ocular metallosis can be electroretinographically divided into four stages: (1) normal ERG; (2) a "neg +" ERG (normal b-wave and increased a-wave); (3) a "neg−" ERG (decreased b-wave and normal or increased a-wave); and (4) extinguished ERG (nonrecordable).[7] Electroretinographic changes appear to be reversible in the neg+ stage and in the early phases of the neg− stage, i.e., when the b-wave reduction is approximately 50 per cent of normal.[7] Thus, the results of ERG testing can affect the decision of whether or not to remove an intraocular piece of metal.

It is interesting that the early receptor potential, a measure of the competence of the photoreceptor outer segments, has been found to be normal in the face of an abnormal ERG. This suggests that the effect on the ERG is at the level of the inner retina and that the photoreceptors are, at least initially, structurally preserved.[9]

Electroretinographic changes have been detected as early as one month after entry of an iron particle and 12 days after entry of a copper particle.[7] These changes may occur before subjective loss of visual acuity or peripheral field. They may also occur before biomicroscopic or ophthalmoscopic evidence of copper deposition is detectable owing to the relatively high ocular toxicity of copper ions. Siderosis, on the other hand, may be detectable on physical examination before ERG changes occur. The explanation for these findings appears to include the fact that iron corrodes more easily than copper in intraocular tissues, whereas copper is apparently more toxic to the tissues if it has access to them.[7]

4.3 REMOVAL OF INTRAOCULAR FOREIGN BODIES

a. Basic Concepts (Table 4–3)

In all cases of retained intraocular foreign bodies, the danger of leaving the foreign body in the eye must be compared with the danger of removing it.

Should any attempt be made to remove the foreign body? As in deciding the relative risk of sympathetic ophthalmia and the possible desirability of enucleation, the ophthalmologist must decide for or against removal of the foreign body after carefully weighing all relevant factors. The contusive, inflammatory, and chemical effects of the initial trauma

Table 4–3. PRINCIPLES OF THERAPY WITH INTRAOCULAR FOREIGN BODIES

1. Close all wounds in the eye.
2. Prevent infection.
3. Clear the ocular media.
4. Remove all vitreous surrounding the foreign body.
5. Remove the foreign body in the least traumatic way.
6. Treat any retinal breaks.

and its probable later inflammatory, chemical, and fibrotic effects must be compared with the risk of detrimental effects from the surgery itself, taking into consideration the possible inability to remove the foreign body atraumatically. In some cases, particularly if the foreign body contains copper, severe inflammatory changes may force the ophthalmologist to consider early surgery despite the inherent dangers of operating on an acutely and severely inflamed eye. Chronic inflammatory, chemical, and fibrotic effects are more or less inevitable, depending largely on the chemical nature of the foreign body and its intraocular location. These effects are especially likely to occur with iron-containing foreign bodies, especially when the iron is in a relatively pure state. Thus, attempts to remove such a retained object should ordinarily be more aggressive. The magnetic characteristics of the iron-containing foreign body would increase the ophthalmologist's willingness to perform the surgery because of the increased ease of magnetic extraction.

The opposite is true concerning a nonmagnetic foreign body such as a copper-containing alloy with low concentration of elemental copper. In such a circumstance the ultimate effects of chalcosis are ordinarily much less severe than in acute copper panophthalmitis and not usually as severe as with a retained iron-containing foreign body. Thus, there would not be as much urgency about removing such a foreign body. However, the advent of intravitreal surgery has made extraction of these foreign bodies much more feasible than in the past.

Foreign objects visible in the anterior segment (Figures 4–12 and 4–13) are usually not difficult to remove, since surgical manipulations can be visually controlled, but the surgical approach should be carefully considered.

A wise surgeon may choose not to undertake extraction of certain

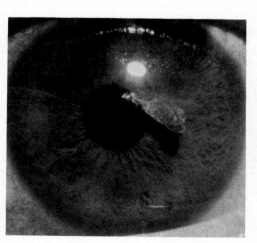

Figure 4–12. A longstanding foreign body in the anterior chamber on the surface of the iris. The point of entry and the nature of the foreign material are unknown, but the object is presumed to be composed of a metal alloy.

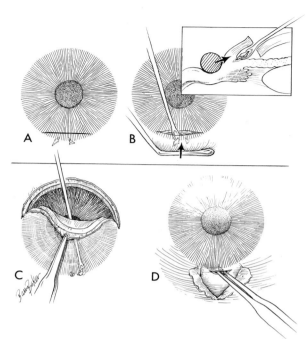

Figure 4–13. Techniques of removing foreign bodies from the anterior chamber. The choice of surgical approach is determined by the size, mobility, and location of the objects and occasionally by the need to perform other intraocular repairs at the time of foreign body removal. (A) and (B) The foreign body is removed through a corneal incision; (C) by a large incision when other intraocular surgery such as lens extraction is required; and (D) through a scleral incision if the foreign body is lodged in the chamber angle.

nonmagnetic foreign bodies that are not visible or are trapped in inflammatory debris. Assuming that the foreign body remains in situ, deterioration of the eye, even with iron-containing foreign bodies, will not invariably occur. Certain foreign bodies may induce enough surrounding encapsulation so that no diffusion of toxic or chemical substances occurs. Total dissolution of the foreign body without induced chemical changes may similarly occur, and spontaneous expulsion of the foreign body from a globe without attendant destruction has also been reported.

If the foreign body is nonmagnetic but visible, pars plana vitrectomy followed by removal through the pars plana (Figure 4–14) or limbus using specialized foreign-body forceps (Figure 4–15) is the best procedure. If the foreign body is invisible but magnetic, ease of extraction is considerably increased.

If the object is small (less than 3 mm in largest diameter) and has rounded rather than ragged contours, magnetic extraction via the portal of entry may be considered. Larger, jagged objects may find the entry site too small for atraumatic passage and may cause added damage to the lens, iris, ciliary body, and cornea during extraction. Therefore, magnetic removal through the pars plana is usually the method of choice after closure of any anterior wound of entry. In most cases, removal of the vitreous through the pars plana should precede any attempt to remove the foreign body.

The patient is prepared for surgery in the routine manner. A consent should be obtained for repair of the ocular wounds, removal of the foreign body and (if necessary) of the lens and vitreous, and retinal detachment repair. Intravenous antibiotics should be started immediately. If a piece of the object from which the foreign body came is available, it should be cultured and its magnetic characteristics evaluated.

It should go without saying that the surgeon should never undertake a procedure without the necessary skills to manage the intraoperative complications that might occur. The practitioner may complete the repair of the entry wounds and then discover that the foreign body is too difficult to remove. In this case, the procedure should be terminated and appropriate referral arranged. With the exception of the injury to the surgeon's ego, no additional harm is likely to be done by this prudent delay in therapy.

b. Removal of Anterior Segment Foreign Bodies

Foreign bodies entering and remaining in the anterior segment of the eye can usually be removed through the wound of entry at the time of primary surgical repair. The presence of blood, fibrin, and uveal prolapse may obscure small foreign bodies that may be identified by bone-free x-ray techniques when suspicion has led to this useful procedure (see Chapter 6).

Fragments of glass, plastic, and other transparent materials are difficult to identify and, being nonmagnetic, must be either visualized or localized with a probe before grasping. Figures 4–13, 4–14, and 4–15 illustrate alternative routes for surgical extraction, the choice of which depends on two factors: (1) the size and nature of the foreign material, and (2) the possibility that other intraocular surgical repairs may necessitate a larger incision at the limbus rather than the small local incision for direct removal of the foreign body from the chamber angle. (For discussion of the management of an intralenticular foreign body see below.)

c. Removal of Magnetic Posterior Segment Foreign Bodies

The magnets available for use include the giant magnet, the permanent hand magnet, the hand electromagnet, the Bronson-Magnion instrument,[10] and the Rare Earth Intraocular Magnet.* The Rare Earth Intraocular Magnet is the only one of the above that can be placed into the eye through a small incision.

Prior to surgery, the surgeon should be convinced that the foreign body is magnetic. One useful technique is to bring the powerful Bronson-Magnion instrument close to the patient while observing the foreign body either directly with an ophthalmoscope or microscope or indirectly with ultrasound. As the instrument is brought closer to the eye, a magnetic foreign body will shift position slightly. As soon as this shift is observed, the magnet should be quickly moved away, as the movement of the foreign body can damage intraocular structures. Another technique is to use the Berman or Bronson-Turner metal locator to find the foreign body, noting that the detecting range for an iron-containing object is about ten times the diameter of the foreign body, whereas the range for a nonmagnetic metal is usually only within one to two times its own diameter (see 4.3c).

Anterior Route (Wound of Entry). The attractive force of any magnet varies with the cube of the distance between it and the foreign body. Consequently, a foreign body, even if magnetic, cannot be extracted anteriorly if it lies too far posteriorly. If the object is weakly magnetic or less than 1 mm in size, similar difficulty may be encountered. The anterior route is dangerous if the foreign body is jagged or greater than 3 mm in size, since intact ocular structures can be irreparably damaged during such an extraction.

A decision of whether to extract a foreign body through the anterior segment requires knowledge of the state of the lens. If the lens is intact and transparent, a posterior route of extraction (through the pars plana) should invariably be used. On the other hand, if the lens has been markedly disrupted, there is much less hesitation about performing an anterior extraction (through the wound of entry). Prior to removing a suspected cataract, the surgeon must be convinced that the lens is, in fact, disrupted. An unwary observer may be misled by the presence of inflammatory debris in the pupillary space and anterior chamber—the result of the original trauma—that may so mimic the appearance of flocculent lens material that only the passage of time will demonstrate the difference between the two. Consequently, lens extraction, whether it is intracapsular, extracapsular, or through the pars plana, should be deferred unless the lens is either obviously disrupted or is observed to become progressively opacified.

Whenever lens extraction is performed, it should be recalled at all times that a perforating injury through the lens produces disruption of the anterior hyaloid face and increases the risk of vitreous loss.

---

*Alcon Surgical Products, Fort Worth, Texas.

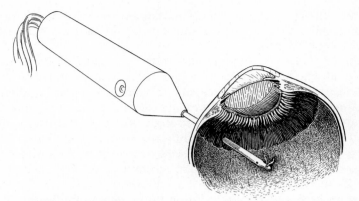

Figure 4–14. Use of the vitrophage in extracting a nonmagnetic foreign body. The foreign body must be small enough to enter the tip of the instrument by suction and be aspirated. Larger foreign bodies can be attracted to the aspiration orifice by suction, and the entire instrument with adherent foreign body removed from the eye. The aperture on the shaft of the handpiece is closed by the surgeon's thumb or forefinger when suction is desired.

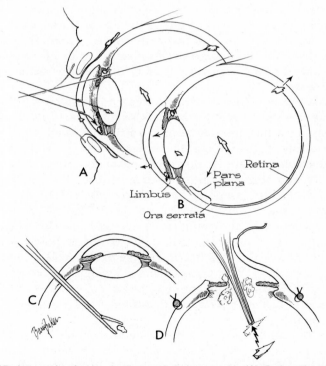

Figure 4–15. Intraocular foreign bodies and their removal. (A) Paths of entry. (B) Usual removal routes. (C) Foreign-body forceps used to grasp nonmagnetic foreign body within the vitreous via incision through pars plana. (D) Removal of magnetic foreign body in the vitreous through limbal incision in an eye with traumatic aphakia. Extraction through the pars plana can also be used in this situation; it is mandatory when the lens is intact and clear (see Figure 4–16).

In performing magnetic extractions via the anterior route, the following technical measures are useful. As in all cases of magnetic foreign-body extraction, the lid speculum and other instruments should be constructed of nonmagnetic materials. The bluntest magnet tip consistent with surgical exposure should be used, since it provides the strongest force. The best available tip is shaped like an acorn. The magnet tip should be brought as close to the foreign body as possible (Figure 4–16). Since magnets have much more strength when cold, intermittent short bursts of current are more effective than prolonged activation, which heats up the magnet. After performing customary procedures such as administration of a preoperative carbonic anhydrase inhibitor and a hyperosmotic agent to soften the eye, the magnet is directed at the original wound of entry, and the current is applied. If the foreign body is magnetic enough or is close enough to the magnet, there should be little difficulty in extracting it through the original wound of entry. Repositioning or excising of prolapsed intraocular contents should then be performed. The wound should be closed with interrupted sutures and the anterior chamber reformed with balanced salt solution if necessary.

Occasionally two directions of pull will be required: one in which the magnet is used to pull the foreign body into the anterior chamber; and one in which the magnet is used to extract the foreign body through a separate, newly created limbal incision. Such a secondary maneuver is useful when the corneal incision is small or self-sealing. The advantages of a new limbal incision are that it can be created under a conjunctival flap and that it can be made regular, without jagged edges, consequently minimizing the danger of uveal or foreign body incarceration.

Posterior Route. When a magnetic foreign body lies in the vitreous cavity or is sitting on the retina, the best approach is through the pars plana. If visible, the location of the foreign body should be carefully drawn with points of reference such as retinal vessels indicated. The

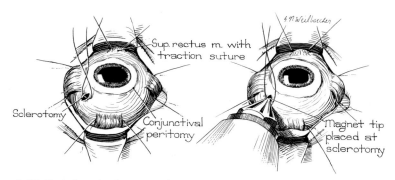

Figure 4–16. Technique for the magnetic extraction of an intraocular foreign body through the pars plana of the ciliary body. In some cases, only one or two traction sutures are needed for adequate exposure, and a total conjunctival peritomy is unnecessary. Note the cone-shaped magnet tip. Ordinarily, the sclerotomy is circumferential, not radial.

wound of penetration is then tightly sutured with 8-0 or 9-0 sutures. A vitrectomy is carried out (see Chapter 10.4c) so that there is no vitreous around the foreign body or in the path that it must pass during removal. This will prevent subsequent traction on the retina and the vitreous base during the extraction.

Once the vitreous has been removed, a plan is made to remove the foreign body in the least traumatic way. The technically simplest method is to place the Bronson-Magnion magnet tip near a sclerotomy that has been prepared to accommodate passage of the foreign body. A preplaced suture should be inserted through the lips of the scleral incision, and the magnet should then be directed at the slightly gaping wound. The surgeon or the assistant should constantly monitor the position of the foreign body using either the indirect ophthalmoscope or the operating microscope.

Even if the magnet is activated correctly, the foreign body may not be removed on the first attempt. There are several possible causes of this, including inappropriate selection of the magnet tip (particularly if a curved tip has been used); entanglement of the foreign body in fibrous and inflammatory debris; and a distant, small, or weakly magnetic foreign body. Extraction of the foreign body often requires extreme patience. Rarely, a small, weakly magnetic foreign body lying distant from the magnet may not be attracted to the extraction site unless a fine, straight blunt probe is inserted into the vitreous through the pars plana incision. Applying the magnet to the handle of the probe then weakly magnetizes the probe. The operator should be wary, however, of an involuntary jerk of the probe when it is magnetized or of inadvertently bumping the probe with the magnet.

Under most circumstances, if the foreign body can be attracted to the sclerotomy, it will cut its own way through the uveal tract, whereupon the surgeon will perceive an audible click or a tactile impression from the magnet tip. Occasionally, however, the foreign body is too dull or the magnet too weak, and the sclerotomy must be enlarged. A straight knife such as a Beaver 52S is excellent for creating a clean, straight incision through the sclera and pars plana, parallel to the limbus. The magnet is then reapplied, and the foreign body is extracted with simultaneous relaxation or all traction and pressure on the globe. The preplaced sclerotomy suture is immediately tied.

While technically more difficult than external magnetic extraction, the use of the Rare Earth Intraocular Magnet (Figure 4–17) provides for a more controlled removal of a magnetic foreign body. When the vitrectomy has been completed, the Intraocular Magnet is introduced through a 20-gauge incision in the pars plana. The tip is slowly advanced toward the foreign body under visualization through the microscope. When it is within the range of attraction, the foreign body will jump onto the tip of the magnet. At this point it should be inspected to ensure that there are

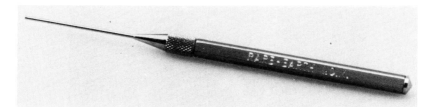

Figure 4–17. Rare Earth Intraocular Magnet. The shaft of this instrument can be placed through a pars plana or limbal incision and then touched to a magnetic foreign body.

no strands of vitreous attached to it and that the retina is not being detached by traction. The instrument is then slowly withdrawn until the foreign body is almost lost from view under the iris. The sclerotomy is then enlarged as necessary and the foreign body removed from the eye. If the object is too large or jagged to be removed through the sclerotomy and the lens has been removed, it may be elevated into the anterior chamber and a separate incision made in the limbus or through the cornea to remove the foreign body.

The advantage of this technique is that the instrument is relatively inexpensive, the extraction can be accomplished through a routine pars plana incision, and the entire extraction can be done under visualization. The magnet is quite strong and can usually pull the foreign body out through the pars plana without dropping it. The disadvantage is that the magnetic substance is continuously activated, and if the foreign body is embedded in the retina it may begin to detach the retina. In such a case, there is no way to cause the magnet to release the foreign body, and a second instrument must be used to "wipe" the foreign body off of the tip.

If a foreign body is embedded in the wall of the eye and overlies the retina and if a direct trans-scleral magnetic extraction is contemplated, precise localization will minimize trauma to the retina. Use of the indirect ophthalmoscope, a Berman or other metal locator, and a high-quality CT scan (Figure 4–18) contributes in large measure to a successful extraction. Transillumination at the time of surgery may also identify precisely the location of the foreign body. For a direct, posterior, trans-scleral extraction, a 360-degree conjunctival peritomy and sling sutures under all of the rectus muscles are required for adequate exposure and atraumatic manipulation and rotation of the globe.

After precise localization of the foreign body, a scleral incision (linear for small foreign bodies, L-shaped for larger ones) is made to the external surface of the uveal tract overlying the foreign body. Under these conditions, ringing the sclerotomy site with diathermy or cryotherapy[2] can be done since postoperative vitreous traction at the wound of exit could produce retinal traction or hole formation (either at the exit site itself or

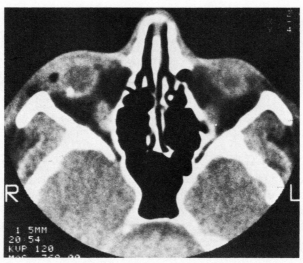

Figure 4–18. CT scan of an intraocular foreign body. The referring physician had closed the entrance wound and noted vitreous and lens material at the wound site. A dense cataract rapidly developed. Plain orbital films taken following the repair disclosed an orbital foreign body, and this CT scan showed that the foreign body was within the globe. At surgery, the foreign body was lifted from a hole in the retina with the Rare Earth Intraocular Magnet and removed through a limbal incision. The postoperative visual acuity was 20/30 after four months.

at a point approximately 180 degrees across the globe). However, what data are available suggest, somewhat to the contrary, that the application of cryotherapy or diathermy over the extraction site may not significantly affect the incidence of either retinal detachment or vitreous hemorrhage.[11]

Because cryoapplications tend to induce uveal vascular engorgement and could thus predispose to hemorrhage, they should be applied *after* removal of the foreign body and closure of the sclerotomy. Vortex radicles should be avoided or, if absolutely necessary, closed with diathermy. Diathermy is usually completed *before* extraction of the foreign body.

After a preplaced suture has been inserted in the lips of the sclerotomy, the magnet is applied; the foreign body either cuts its own way through the uveal tract or is extracted after a uveal stab incision is made; the preplaced suture is closed. Under most circumstances, this series of maneuvers is sufficient. However, with the likelihood of significant vitreous traction, the choice may be to extract the foreign body through a lamellar scleral bed, prepared as in a routine scleral undermining procedure for repair of retinal detachment. The diathermized or cryotherapized scleral bed is then buckled inward to reduce traction on the underlying retina (Figure 4–19). An alternative technique is to extract the foreign body through full-thickness sclera, followed by a buckling procedure with an external element.

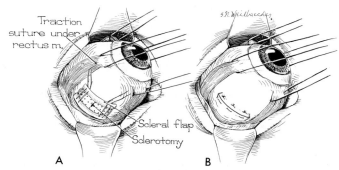

Figure 4–19. Technique for removal of an intraocular foreign body through the choroid. (A) Undermined scleral flaps are dissected, and the lamellar scleral bed is pretreated with diathermy or cryotherapy. (B) After foreign body extraction, the scleral bed is buckled inward.

d. Removal of Nonmagnetic Foreign Bodies

Surgical maneuvers to remove nonmagnetic foreign bodies are consider-ably more difficult and potentially more disruptive to the vitreous than removal of magnetic objects because of the intravitreal manipulations involved. If the foreign body is lodged in the wall of the eye, direct trans-scleral extraction should be performed as in the previously described procedure for magnetic extraction. To minimize vitreous trauma, the sclerotomy must directly and precisely overlie the foreign body. If locali-zation has been correct and precise (within 1 mm), the scleral incision, performed in the manner already described, will provide direct visualiz-ation of the foreign body. If it lies within the wall of the eye, it can be simply lifted out of its resting place with forceps. Closure of the sclerot-omy, with or without simultaneous scleral buckling, should be completed as detailed previously.

If the foreign body lies intravitreally or sits on the retina, a pars plana vitrectomy should be carried out to remove all vitreous from around the foreign body and from the path of removal.

There are several devices useful for removing the foreign body. Intravitreal foreign body forceps (Neubauer, Thorpe, Greishaber) are among those available. The best appears to be the Greishaber diamond-coated forceps, as they are easy to manipulate and grip the foreign body well. Small intravitreal cryoprobes are useful for holding foreign bodies that contain vegetable material and for retrieving a lens nucleus if it is dislocated posteriorly during lensectomy. Alternatively, a needle or pick can be used to nudge the object into the suction port of the vitrectomy probe, and the foreign body can then be elevated into the anterior chamber where it can be grasped through a limbal or corneal incision.

e. Removal of Intralenticular Foreign Bodies

When a magnetic foreign body comes to rest in the lens, a cataract may or may not occur. Furthermore, siderosis of the globe may or may not occur; in fact, the lens appears to retard the dissemination of toxic iron to other portions of the eye. Tiny foreign bodies are best left in the lens, whether or not they are magnetic. It has been noted that small or medium-sized magnetic foreign bodies should be removed along the entrance pathway as atraumatically as possible, with a magnet just strong enough to perform the extraction.[12] Tears in the lens capsule may seal without causing widespread cataractous changes if they are 2 mm in size or smaller (Figure 4–20). Therefore, the lens should not be removed in such cases

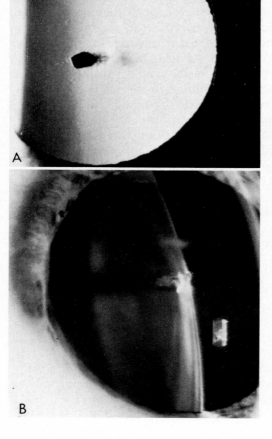

Figure 4–20. An intralenticular metallic foreign body present in the lens for ten days. If a cataract does not develop, such a foreign body may be allowed to remain within the lens. In this case, visual acuity was 20/30 at the time the photographs were taken. (A) Foreign body seen with retroillumination. (B) Foreign body seen with direct illumination.

unless it is observed to progressively opacify. Large foreign bodies, manipulation of which will cause a diffuse cataract, should be managed by cryoextraction of the entire lens with the foreign body within it.

4.4 REMOVAL OF INTRAORBITAL MAGNETIC, NONMAGNETIC, ORGANIC, AND INORGANIC FOREIGN BODIES

Foreign bodies often remain within the orbit for a considerable length of time (up to many years) without eliciting troublesome symptoms or signs. This is true of most metal foreign bodies, including iron, steel, lead, and aluminum; however, copper-containing objects may incite a purulent inflammation similar in some respects to the reaction induced by intraocular copper particles. Intraorbital plastic, glass, and stone are generally quiescent.

A different situation is observed with intraorbital retention of organic foreign bodies, particularly those of wood. After an initial quiescent period of considerable variation in duration (days to years), the following complications often arise: granuloma, orbital cellulitis, orbital abscess, osteomyelitis, periostitis, or chronically draining fistula (through the conjunctiva or through the palpebral skin). In these situations, the foreign body is frequently occult owing to its posterior location within the orbit and its relative radiolucency. Correct interpretation of the inflammatory signs requires careful history-taking and physical examination as well as a variety of diagnostic adjuncts, most notably CT scanning (see Chapter 6).

If and when symptoms due to intraocular retention of a foreign body are finally manifested, the interval between injury and onset of disability is often so great (and the original incident seemingly so trivial) that the patient may fail to tell the physician about the original trauma. As in many types of ophthalmic injuries, only particular suspicion of a foreign body leads to proper interrogation of the patient.

Most large foreign bodies entering the orbit slide between the eye and the orbital bony walls (Figures 4–21, 4–22, and 4–23). Fortunately, severe injury to the eye is rare in such accidents, unless the foreign body has unusual momentum, e.g., a bullet. However, immediate direct trauma to important structures of the muscle cone may occasionally result in paresis of an extraocular muscle or damage to the optic nerve. If a foreign body strikes the apex of the orbit, a blind, anesthetic, and immobile globe may result. Rarely, the foreign body will traverse the orbit and penetrate into a paranasal sinus, the nose, or the intracranial space. Under these circumstances, serious infection and other damage can occur, up to and including death.

Treatment of most intraorbital foreign bodies should be conservative and expectant unless any of the following occurs: severe inflammatory signs (e.g., from abscess, cellulitis, fistula), compressive effects on the eye

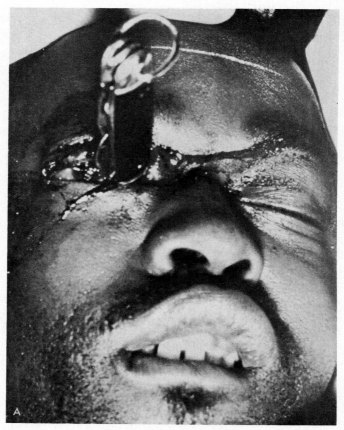

Figure 4–21. (A) A 35-year-old man with a penknife embedded to the hilt in the right orbit. There was no light perception in the right eye, and total ophthalmoplegia had occurred, although the globe itself was intact.

Illustration continued on opposite page

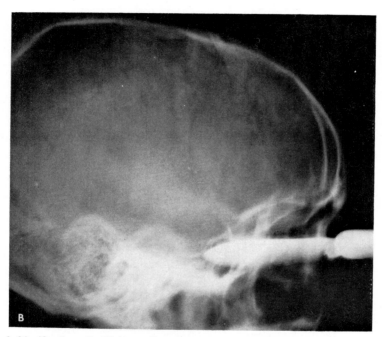

Figure 4–21. *(Continued).* (B) X-ray film showing the tip of the blade next to the sphenoid sinus. The knife was removed by simultaneous right frontal craniotomy and orbital exploration. The knife had not entered the dura but had severed the optic nerve and the medial rectus muscle. Except for ophthalmoplegia and loss of vision in the damaged eye, the patient's recovery was uneventful. Any penetrating injury of the orbit should suggest the possibility of intracranial involvement. (This case was reported previously; photographs published with permission of the authors: Bard LA, Jarrett WH: Intracranial complications of penetrating orbital injuries. Arch Ophthalmol, *71*:332–343, 1964.)

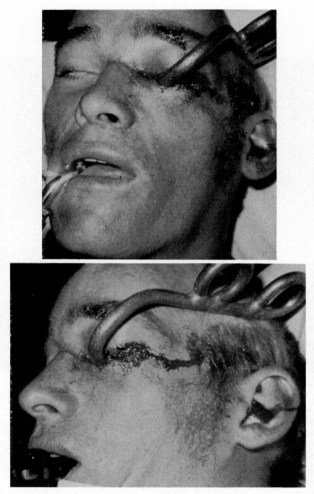

Figure 4–22. Injury similar to the case pictured in Figure 4–21. This meat hook injury of the left orbit caused no damage to the globe itself, although the tip of the hook entered the frontal lobe in the anterior cranial fossa. There was also damage to the optic nerve with loss of light perception, but there were no intracranial sequelae from this injury once the meat hook was removed. (Photographs published through the courtesy of William M. Aden, M.D.)

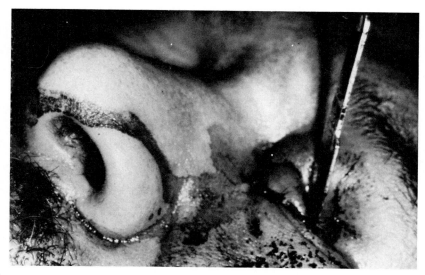

Figure 4–23. Intraorbital foreign body. A friend of the patient thrust this steak knife into the patient's orbit. The patient pulled off the plastic handle in his attempt to remove the knife. When removed in the operating room, no ocular injury was found. The knife had passed inferior to the globe, through the infraorbital fissure, and into the infratemporal fossa. The visual acuity two days after the injury was 20/20.

(e.g., from orbital pseudotumor), or communication between the orbit and a paranasal sinus or the intracranial space. Surgical removal requires careful localization by all available techniques, because damage to important intraconal structures is inadvertently induced all too easily. In addition, many foreign bodies, especially organic and wooden ones, will fragment during removal attempts, leaving behind splinters that will propagate the inflammatory process. Blunt dissection, careful hemostasis, and excellent lighting and exposure will aid in atraumatic removal of all of the splinters. Bayonet, alligator-jaw, and other specialized extraction forceps are extremely helpful.

The surgical approach to the foreign body will depend on its location within the orbit. If the object lies anterior to the equator of the globe, a direct approach through the wound of entry or fistulous track may be considered. A separate subperiosteal incision in a quadrant nearest the foreign body has been employed successfully, and a standard lateral orbitotomy is also useful. Occasionally, a transfrontal craniotomy is necessary. The necessity of using a magnet to assist in the removal of magnetic intraorbital foreign bodies is sufficiently evident not to require elaboration. A foreign body lodged simultaneously in the orbit and in either a paranasal sinus or the intracranial space requires the cooperation of an ENT surgeon or neurosurgeon in a team approach.

References

1. Goldberg MF: Management of posterior segment intraocular foreign bodies. J Miss State Med Assoc 11:149–158, 1970.
2. Havener WH, Gloeckner SL: Atlas of Diagnostic Techniques and Treatment of Intraocular Foreign Bodies. St. Louis, C. V. Mosby Co, 1969.
3. Duke-Elder S, MacFaul PA: System of Ophthalmology. Vol. XIV, Injuries. St. Louis, C. V. Mosby Co, 1972.
4. Jones LT: Tear-sac foreign bodies. Am J Ophthalmol 60:111–113, 1965.
5. Guy LP: Use of Berman locator in removal of magnetic intraocular foreign bodies. Arch Ophthalmol 36:540–550, 1946.
6. Percival SPB: A decade of intraocular foreign bodies. Br J Ophthalmol 56:454–461, 1972.
7. Knave B: Electroretinography in eyes with retained intraocular metallic foreign bodies. Acta Ophthalmol Suppl 100, 1969.
8. Beckerman BL: Intraocular foreign body extraction in early chalcosis. Arch Ophthalmol 87:444–446, 1972.
9. Sieving PA, Fishman GA, Alexander KR, Goldberg MF: Early receptor potential measurements in human ocular siderosis. Arch Ophthalmol 101:1716–1720, 1983.
10. Bronson NR II: Practical characteristics of ophthalmic magnets. Arch Ophthalmol 79:22–27, 1968.
11. Percival SPB: Late complications from posterior segment intraocular foreign bodies with particular reference to retinal detachment. Br J Ophthalmol 56:462–468, 1972.
12. Keeney AH: Intralenticular foreign bodies. Arch Ophthalmol 86:499–501, 1971.

CHAPTER

5

Burns of the Eye and Adnexa

5.1 CHEMICAL BURNS

a. *Common Causes*

Burns of the eye caused by alkali or acid are among the most urgent ocular emergencies (Table 5–1). Because of the more rapid penetration of alkaline materials into the cornea and anterior chamber, the results of alkali burns are frequently more disastrous than those of burns caused by acids.[1]

Acid burns cause their damage within the first few hours. Thereafter their damage is less progressive and less penetrating. Acids quickly precipitate tissue proteins and thus set up physical barriers against tissue penetration. Subsequent buffering of the acids by surrounding tissue proteins tends to localize the damage at the area of contact. (The exceptions are burns from hydrofluoric acid and from acids containing heavy metals. Strong acids such as these rapidly penetrate the cornea, kill the endothelium, and ultimately give rise to a retrocorneal membrane and a vascularized, opaque cornea.)

Such favorable factors unfortunately do not apply to alkali burns. Alkalis combine with the lipids of cellular membranes and thus produce

Table 5–1. STEPS IN EVALUATION AND TREATMENT OF ALKALI BURNS

 1. History.
 2. Visual acuity.
 3. Determination of conjunctival pH.
 4. Initial lavage and removal of particulate debris (this step should take place virtually at the same time as the first three steps).
 5. Determination of intraocular pressure.
 6. Paracentesis of anterior chamber.
 7. Prolonged lavage (1 liter for each eye).
 8. Cycloplegia.
 9. Topical antibiotics.
10. Treatment of elevated intraocular pressure as necessary.
11. Steroids.
12. Evaluation of nonocular injuries.

total disruption of cells with softening of the tissue. Additional alkali can therefore penetrate rapidly, and the effect may continue for days. In the cornea, severe disruption of the stromal mucopolysaccharides occurs, resulting in rapid opacification (Figures 5–1 and 5–2). The inferior cornea is generally affected the most, as the Bell's phenomenon reflexively protects the eye. Strong alkalis cause ischemia and coagulation necrosis of conjunctiva and sclera; in addition, if bits of alkaline debris are allowed to remain in contact with the globe, perforation may result because of coagulation through conjunctiva, sclera, choroid, and retina.[2] Coagulation

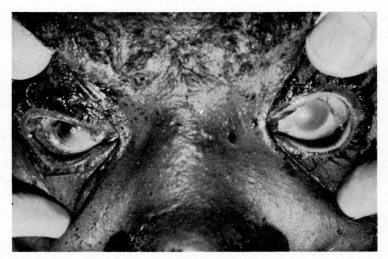

Figure 5–1. Lye burns of the eyes and lids. Pearly opacity of the cornea and blanching of the conjunctiva are poor prognostic signs. Ultimately, the left eye may be lost from keratitis sicca, perforated descemetocele, or infection. Salvage of such eyes by topical use of collagenase inhibitors, judicious use of steroids, and hydrophilic lenses is possible, but useful vision for this patient's left eye would require eventual penetrating keratoplasty or, more likely of long-range success, a keratoprosthesis with scleral overlay graft to reinforce the cornea.

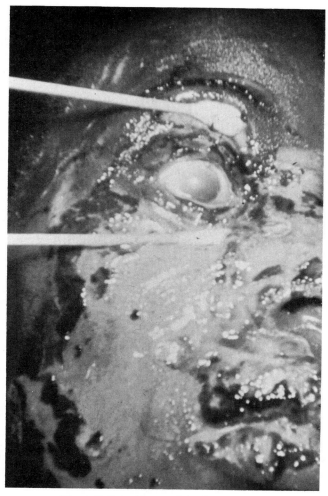

Figure 5–2. Lye burns of the face and eye.

of the trabecular structures can result in late glaucoma. Destruction of the tear-producing cells of the conjunctiva and obliteration of the tear ducts draining the lacrimal glands can result in a severe dry eye syndrome.

The extent of damage is evaluated based on the severity of corneal opacification (as measured by the ability to see details of the anterior chamber and iris) and the degree of perilimbal ischemia (as measured by the blanching of the episcleral vessels).[3] Of these, the amount of perilimbal blanching appears to be the most important prognostic sign.

Alkali burns caused by lye (NaOH, or KOH), fresh lime (CaO), and ammonia are the ones most frequently observed in this country. The damage is related more to the alkalinity than to the cation. The extent of permanent injury is determined not only by the nature and concentration of the chemical but also by the time lapse preceding decontamination. Elevation of aqueous pH can be detected after only 15 seconds of corneal contact with strong alkalis. Unless the eye is copiously irrigated within moments, it may eventually be lost. Because of the extreme importance of speed in the treatment of these injuries, the physician must be ready to begin treatment immediately. The necessary equipment should be readily available at all times in eye emergency rooms. The general steps involved in the evaluation and treatment of these injuries are given in Table 5–1.

The initial rapid rise in intraocular pressure after alkali burns is attributed to shrinkage of the outer coats of the eye, whereas the later elevation of tension is thought to be from intraocular release of prostaglandins[4] and ultimately from sclerosis of outflow channels.[3] In acid burns, hydrogen ions enter into the anterior chamber, causing a release of prostaglandins. The resulting pressure rise may be blocked by indomethacin.[5]

Riot control agents such as tear gas and mace do not commonly cause permanent ocular damage in the low concentrations that usually reach the eyes, although eyes lost from such agents have been reported.[6] Eyes traumatized by tear gas or mace should be managed like other chemically burned eyes (often with concomitant contusion injuries), for there is no specific therapy.[6, 7] *The examiner should also be on the lookout for perforating ocular injuries and intraocular foreign bodies projected into the eye from foreign matter contained in tear gas pens or aerosol sprays.*[8]

Injuries to the eyes from sparklers or flares are attributable to magnesium hydroxide and should be managed as chemical (as distinguished from thermal) burns.[9]

In past decades, mustard gas, nitrogen mustard, and lewisite (treated by dimercaprol) were the most common vesicant war gases causing injury to the eye.

b. Medical Treatment

With the rare exception of chemicals that react violently with water, the immediate treatment of chemical burns must be copious irrigation of the eyes, using the most readily available source of water: shower, spigot, drinking fountain, hose, or bathtub. The lids must be held apart manually or with retractors (Figure 5–3), because severe orbicularis spasm and lid closure may otherwise prevent the eye from receiving the beneficial effect of the irrigation. Particulate chemical matter should be promptly removed with cotton swabs or forceps, the lids should be singly and doubly everted (see Figure 4–5), and the fornices of the conjunctival sac should be swept

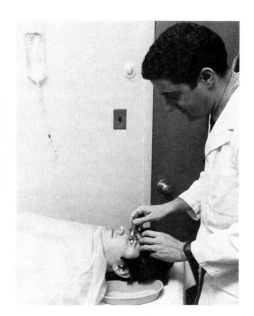

Figure 5–3. Proper technique for irrigation of the eye following a chemical burn. The lids are being retracted with a Desmarres retractor to expose the fornices. Normal saline is being used as the irrigant. (From Deutsch TA, Feller DB: Injuries of the eye, the lids and the orbit. In *The Management of Trauma* (Fourth Edition). Zuidema GD, et al, eds; Philadelphia, WB Saunders Co, in press.)

with cotton applicators. Topical anesthetic eyedrops and local anesthetic injections by the O'Brien technique (see Figure 2–5) may be required for these procedures if blepharospasm is severe.

After initial lavage, early use of topical anesthetics will greatly facilitate further emergency measures by easing the patient's discomfort. If paracentesis is not elected as the next step, irrigation should be continued for a minimum of 1 liter for each eye with a reservoir of normal saline connected to an intravenous tubing set (see Figure 5–3). If the nature of the chemical irritant is unknown, the use of pH paper touched to the involved tissue will show whether the chemical is acidic or basic. The same paper can be used after copious irrigation to make certain that the pH is back within the normal range.[10]

The use of neutralizing solutions is not generally feasible for the treatment of chemical burns, because these agents are rarely immediately available. A strong case can be made for hypertonic buffer (monobasic potassium phosphate and dibasic sodium phosphate prepared in 0.5 molar concentration with respect to the phosphate) in the therapy of both acid and alkali burns,[11] but no buffer is as available as water. There are only a few specific antidotes of proven value in treating ocular burns from common chemicals. For example, fresh lime, mortar, and plaster (all of which contain calcium hydroxide) are removed with greater ease by the use of 0.01M solution of neutral sodium edathamil (EDTA)[12]; cocaine solution is effective with iodine burns[13]; and sodium chloride is the optimal irrigation solution for silver nitrate burns.[13] However, since time is a vital factor, *precious moments should not be wasted while a search is made for specific antidotes.*

After lavage, strong cycloplegics (atropine, scopolamine, or homatropine) are instilled to minimize iris adhesions to the lens. It is sometimes helpful to start treatment with topical corticosteroids, which may include a sterile hypopyon when there have been extensive corneal burns from alkali, to reduce iridocyclitis. The use of corticosteroids is controversial, however, and the patient must be monitored carefully if they are used. The danger of ulceration does not appear to be increased by steroid therapy during the first week of treatment.[14] Medroxyprogesterone has also been reported to favorably influence the healing of alkali burns, but subsequent evidence has cast doubt on these data.[15]

Cysteine (0.2M solution, 1 to 2 drops every two hours), acetylcysteine (Mucomyst, 20% solution, same dose regimen), or other collagenase inhibitors may prevent loss of corneal stroma by the action of collagenase liberated from injured corneal and conjunctival epithelium.[16] The use of such agents, however, has not gained clinical acceptance. The therapeutic use of a soft bandage–type contact lens in combination with cysteine solution reportedly has been beneficial in at least one clinical series.[17] Other authors advocate collagenase inhibition by calcium edetate[18] or penicillamine 0.15M.[19]

Recently, it has been observed that the aqueous of animals subjected to severe alkali burns is relatively scorbutic. This has led investigators to study the use of ascorbic acid in the treatment of these injuries.[20] Both ascorbate and citrate have been found experimentally to reduce the rate of ulceration in alkali burns. A clinical trial is underway to determine whether this treatment is clinically efficacious.

Moderate and severe chemical burns by alkali or acid may lead to scarring of both the palpebral and bulbar conjunctiva, with resultant adhesions between the lids and the globe (symblepharon). The use of a scleral contact lens or other conformer fitted into the conjunctival fornices may be of some help in reducing this scarring, which can be a late complication of great severity.

Besides corneal damage, cataract and glaucoma are common sequelae of severe chemical burns—alkali burns in particular. Most eyes so affected have had hypopyon in the acute state after the burn.[17] Any severe alkali burn of the cornea should lead to the presumption (and appropriate treatment) of secondary glaucoma, particularly if tonometry cannot be performed.[21]

Since toxic chemicals can be aspirated into the lungs rather easily when they initially strike the face, the alert physician will inspect the larynx and pharynx and will be prepared to manage acute obstruction of the airway.

c. Surgical Treatment

On the basis of experimental evidence, immediate paracentesis seems to be indicated in moderately severe and severe alkali burns.[22] The data suggest that the value of external lavage in lowering aqueous pH is relatively small, but pH is significantly lowered by paracentesis alone and is further lowered by re-formation of the anterior chamber with phosphate buffer. Thus, on the basis of experimental evidence, paracentesis for the management of severe alkali burns seems advisable; sterile phosphate buffer or other irrigant solutions may be beneficial in reducing intraocular damage even several hours after the alkali burn.

If large areas of conjunctiva are necrotic, particularly if there is contact between denuded bulbar and palpebral conjunctival surfaces, symblepharon may occur. Mucous membrane grafts may be necessary to prevent this. When the cornea fails to epithelialize or heals with major vascularization, conjunctival transplantation may be helpful.[23]

In rare instances, severe chemical burns of the cornea are treated by emergency lamellar[24] or penetrating corneal grafts to salvage the eye when corneal destruction is so extensive that eventual perforation of the cornea is inevitable. Such grafts will not be optically clear, healing will be prolonged, and glaucoma and cataract may complicate the challenge of saving the eye for useful vision at a later date.

5.2 THERMAL BURNS

a. Principal Types

Lid Burns. Thermal burns of the lids are treated in much the same way as thermal burns elsewhere in the body. Marked edema and tissue necrosis are usually present (Figure 5–4), making examination of the globe dependent on the use of lid retractors. Exposure to flame rarely involves the cornea and globe. Reflex lid closure, Bell's phenomenon of upward rotation of the eyes, and rapid reflex movements of the head protect the eye so that the burns usually involve only the lids.

Partial or full-thickness skin loss in the lid is particularly disabling, since ectropion almost invariably occurs from subsequent scarring (Figure 5–5). Although the cosmetic blemish is disfiguring, the attendant possibilities of chronic epiphora, exposure keratitis, trichiasis, and corneal ulceration or perforation are obviously of far greater functional importance.

Contact Burns. Contact burns, such as those caused by flying tobacco ash or molten metal, can produce permanent scarring. This is particularly true of burns caused by glass and metals, such as iron, that have high melting points (1,200° C).[13] Metals with lower melting points (lead, tin, or zinc, which melt at 1000° C or below) do much less damage, and although an external cast of the eye can be formed by such molten metals, permanent visual disability is exceptional.

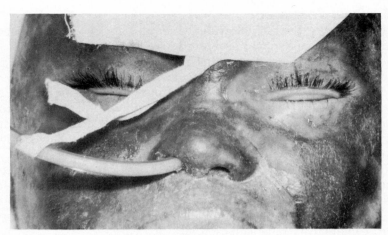

Figure 5–4. The patient is shown shortly after sustaining severe thermal burns of the face. Note that there is bilateral entropion of the lower lids and ectropion of the upper lids.

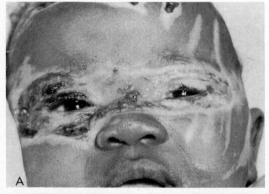

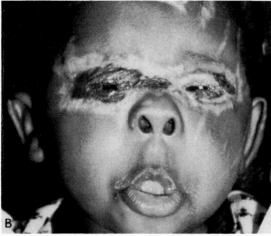

Figure 5–5. Second- and third-degree burns primarily affecting the lids. (A) The patient had fallen against a radiator. In this case, a full-thickness harlequin-type skin graft was used to cover the denuded periocular areas and the nasal bridge. (B) Same patient two years later, showing the severe sequelae of the original burn and an unfavorable surgical result.

b. Medical Treatment

As in all cases of burns, the treatment of shock and the control of infection are of primary importance in treating severe thermal burns that include the ocular structures. Intravenous fluids and use of a transnasal catheter for feedings are sometimes indicated with severe facial burns.

For partial-thickness burns of the eyelids, an antibiotic ointment with a sterile dressing is customarily used, but for minimal burns no dressing is necessary. Frequent application of moist or lubricated dressings, avoidance of extensive debridement in the early stages, prevention of secondary infection, and protection of the cornea are the chief factors in management. The use of prophylactic antibiotics for partial-thickness burns of the eyelids is the same as that for burns elsewhere on the body, except that only ophthalmic preparations may be used on or near the eye. The role of topical steroids remains controversial, for they may enhance glaucoma and, in the presence of corneal destruction, may increase the likelihood of secondary infection and augment the ulcerogenic effect of collagenase. Yet, in reduction of symblepharon (especially if the corneal lesion is not serious), steroids undoubtedly play a beneficial role. Furthermore, control of *intraocular* inflammation is often a prime concern.

For temporary protection of severely burned eyelids, a piece of cellophane can be most useful.[25] It is also useful for patients with marked exophthalmos, severe conjunctival hemorrhage or chemosis, and traumatic absence of the eyelids (Figure 5–6). The plastic film is cut into pieces large enough to cover the entire orbit from the forehead to the cheek. These rectangular pieces (approximately 4 × 6 inches) can be gas-

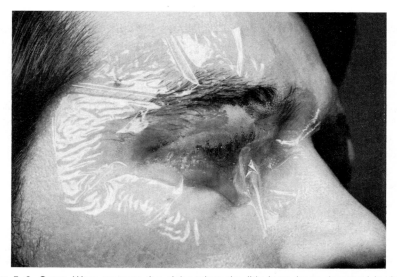

Figure 5–6. Saran Wrap protects the globe when the lids have been damaged by burns, mechanical trauma, or seventh-nerve paralysis. A moist chamber is established.

autoclaved in individual packages. A thin layer of petrolatum ointment is
then applied to the skin around the orbit, and the sterile wrap is placed
over the area to be protected. The plastic will adhere to the skin both by
static charge and by surface tension, thus creating a moisture-proof cover
for the exposed cornea, conjunctiva, and/or damaged eyelids. Small
droplets of moisture will appear on the inner surface of the plastic, and if
these become excessive, several small holes can be punched in the plastic
to allow some evaporation and exchange of gases while retaining sufficient
moisture for the cornea and conjunctiva. In milder burn cases, artificial
tears or a bland ophthalmic ointment may be sufficient protection.

c. Surgical Treatment

In full-thickness burns of the lids, minimization of scarring and ectropion
formation are obtained through full-thickness skin grafting at the earliest
possible time.[13, 26, 27] The host area should be initially debrided of devital-
ized tissues and exuberant granulations. Ideally, the graft should be
performed on the day of injury. If this is not done or if a tarsorrhaphy (to
minimize cicatricial shrinkage) is impossible because of extensive loss of
lid tissue, the cornea must be protected by a moist orbital environment,
as described previously. A soft contact lens will not remain moist in the
absence of functional eyelids and is therefore not helpful in these cases.

As soon as possible, more definitive corneal protection must be
obtained, possibly from a thin conjunctival flap.[28, 29] The globe that is
protected by a hood conjunctival flap must also be lubricated with artificial
tears or protected by cellophane until lid reconstruction is completed.
Since removal of such a flap after the lids have been reconstructed is
readily accomplished with accompanying restoration of vision (assuming
no central corneal scarring), there should be no hesitation in performing
this operation if the patient is medically stable enough to be brought to
the operating room. A thick conjunctival flap will frequently retract and
is therefore inferior to the thin variety.

If initial skin grafting to the lids is impossible, spontaneous separation
of the skin slough occurs after about three weeks, at which time definitive
grafting can be performed. If the underlying bed is covered by exuberant
granulations, these should be excised, along with any necrotic tissue,
down to a smooth, firm base. Grafting can then commence.[13, 26, 30] Once
granulations have begun, split-thickness grafts are more advisable and
safer than full-thickness ones. Such grafts (of 0.005-inch thickness) are
conveniently obtained from the medial surface of the upper arm.

Lid burns of both full and partial thickness often are complicated by
profuse discharge and crusting when treatment does not begin until one
or more days after injury. Wet antibiotic dressings should be changed
numerous times a day. The mild debridement produced by wet gauze is

usually sufficient to remove the crusts. Dilute solutions of hydrogen peroxide may also be used to gently debride the crusts.

Symblepharon formation may occur if opposing portions of the bulbar and palpebral conjunctiva are burned. Immediate conjunctival (from the contralateral eye) or buccal mucous membrane grafting is the most effective therapy against symblepharon formation. The Castroviejo electric mucotome, when properly used with lip mucosa ballooned "on the stretch" by submucosal injection of saline solution, is by far the best way to get thin donor tissue.[31] Whereas the graft would be excessively pink if it were full-thickness, it will be virtually transparent if obtained with a mucotome.[26]

Corneal burns are treated with topical cycloplegics and antibiotics. Topical steroids probably minimize inflammation and scarring, but ulceration and perforation are possible steroid-induced complications. There is rarely enough tissue loss to justify emergency corneal grafting.

5.3 RADIATION BURNS

a. Ultraviolet and Infrared Burns

Ultraviolet light–induced keratitis is discussed in Chapter 7. Ultraviolet irradiation rarely damages the lens and does so only if the intensity has been extremely high; the retina is unaffected. Chronic actinic keratoconjunctivitis and its relationship to pinguecula, marginal corneal dellen, and the pathogenesis of pterygia are discussed thoroughly elsewhere.[32]

Infrared flash burns are usually of little consequence; the lids develop an immediate, temporary erythema, but the eye itself is usually unharmed. However, prolonged exposure to the shorter wavelengths of infrared is responsible for the development of heat cataracts. Glassblowers and metal-furnace stokers, who in the past were improperly protected from the radiation, have developed cataracts after many years of such employment. The lens is susceptible to damage because of its lack of blood supply (heat is not rapidly removed) and because injured lens cells cannot be replaced, as can cells of other exposed tissues.

b. Radiation Cataracts

Cataracts can be a late result of ionizing radiation of various types; high-speed neutrons from cyclotron exposure and atomic blasts are the most typical source. Beta radiation will also cause cataracts if the eye is exposed to excessive doses.[33, 34]

Patients who receive radiation of the head and neck in the treatment of cancer may develop cataracts as well. The minimal cataractogenic dose from x-rays is approximately 500 to 800 rads at the surface of the lens.

The lens is most vulnerable to x-ray exposure in utero and probably least vulnerable in old age. A latency period of 6 to 24 months (and up to 12 years) exists. The higher the dose, the shorter the latency. The latencies with gamma rays and neutrons are of similar length.

Electric current can, on occasion, induce lens changes. The pathogenesis remains unclear. A latency period of months to years exists. When an electrical injury is sustained, especially by the head, the pupil should be dilated within a few weeks after injury and the lens examined for the presence of characteristic vacuoles of prognostic importance.[35] Diathermy also can be cataractogenic via its thermal properties. Ultraviolet and grenz rays damage the lens only if their intensity has been high (at least high enough to damage the cornea).

For details on ultrasonic, electrical, and various radiational injuries to the eye, the reader is referred elsewhere,[36, 37] since these are relatively uncommon and do not require special emergency room management.

c. Solar Viewing

Visible light can cause flash blindness with temporary retinal dysfunction or moderate to severe degrees of retinal edema and atrophy, depending on the light intensity and length of exposure. Many affected persons develop great anxiety from such untoward exposures. An eye with a previously abnormal macula (degenerative, edematous) will suffer prolonged and more severe effects from exposure to bright light than will a normal eye. Unprotected viewing of the sun (as during a solar eclipse) can cause irreversible damage to the macula (Figure 5–7). Visible rays and

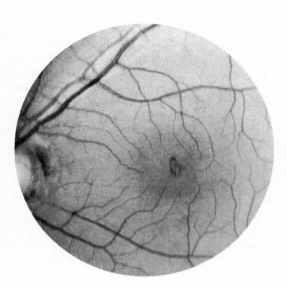

Figure 5–7. Solar maculopathy. A macular burn was sustained by this patient, a self-avowed "sun worshipper."

the short infrared rays are refracted onto the macula, with resultant burning. The immediate decrease in visual acuity may become permanent, but normal acuity is sometimes re-established. The macular lesion occurring in young military men, and known as foveomacular retinitis, may be caused by a self-inflicted solar burn.[38]

d. Laser Accidents

Industrial laser accidents are contributing to an increasing number of ocular injuries.[39] These accidents can cause macular burns, which are sudden and tragic (Figure 5–8).

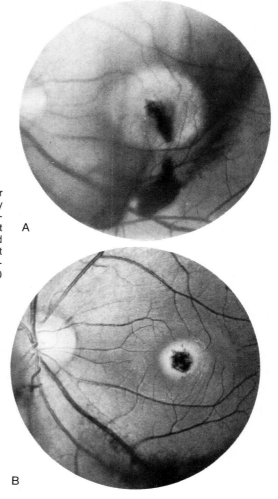

Figure 5–8. (A) and (B) Industrial laser macular burn. This patient accidently gazed into the aiming beam of an industrial laser, resulting in an instant decrease in visual acuity. (Reprinted with permission from Goldberg MF, et al: Macular hole caused by a 589-nanometer dye laser operating for 10 nanoseconds. Retina 3:40–44, 1983.)

A

B

e. *Preventive Measures*

Since no emergency or other treatment is successful for radiation burns of the retina or lens, prophylaxis is all important. Ultraviolet burns can be prevented by ordinary spectacle crown glass or by window glass, since they absorb these rays. Avoidance of short-wave infrared burns has been largely accomplished via mechanization of furnaces. Lead screens absorb much of the dangerous x-, gamma, and neutron radiation.

Prevention of solar eclipse blindness is *never* accomplished by simply holding tinted glass or untreated photographic film in front of the eyes. Only the visible rays, and not the infrared, are thereby diminished. Public education is necessary around the time of each solar eclipse to prevent the needless tragedy of eclipse blindness.

References

1. Escapini H: Trauma to the cornea. In *The Cornea: World Congress*. King JH Jr, McTigue JW, eds; London, Butterworth & Co, 1965, 300–315.
2. Smith RE, Conway B: Alkali retinopathy. Arch Ophthalmol 94:81–84, 1976.
3. Lemp MA: Annual review: cornea and sclera. Arch Ophthalmol 92:158–170, 1974.
4. Paterson CA, Pfister RR: Intraocular pressure changes after alkali burns. Arch Ophthalmol 91:211–218, 1974.
5. Paterson CA, Eakins KE, Paterson E, Jenkins RM II, Ishikawa R: The ocular hypertensive response following experimental acid burns in the rabbit eye. Invest Ophthalmol Vis Sci 18:67–74, 1979.
6. Leopold IH, Lieberman TW: Chemical injuries of the cornea. Fed Proc 30:92–95, 1971.
7. Leopold IH, Maylath FR: Intraocular penetration of cortisone and its effectiveness against experimental corneal burns. Am J Ophthalmol 35:1125–1134, 1952.
8. Borer MJ, Stewart LD: Tear gas spray injury: an unusual case. Ann Ophthalmol 4:783–786, 1972.
9. Harris LS, Cohn K, Galin MA: Alkali injury from fireworks. Ann Ophthalmol 3:849–851, 1971.
10. Tenzel RR: Trauma and burns. Int Ophthalmol Clin 10(1):55–69, 1970.
11. Poser E: Emergency treatment of chemical injuries. Ill Med J 127:161–162, 1965.
12. Grant WM: *Toxicology of the Eye*. (Second Edition). Springfield, Ill, Charles C Thomas Co, 1974.
13. Duke-Elder S, MacFaul PA: *System of Ophthalmology*. Vol. XIV, *Injuries*. St. Louis, C. V. Mosby Co, 1972.
14. Donshik PC, Berman MB, Dohlman CH, Gage J, Rose J: Effect of topical corticosteroids on ulceration in alkali-burned corneas. Arch Ophthalmol 96:2117–2120, 1978.
15. Lass JH, Campbell RC, Rose J, Foster CS, Dohlman CH: Medroxyprogesterone on corneal ulceration. Its effect after alkali burns on rabbits. Arch Ophthalmol 99:673–676, 1981.
16. Brown SI, Weller CA: The pathogenesis and treatment of collagenase-induced diseases of the cornea. Trans Am Acad Ophthalmol Otolaryngol 74:375–383, 1970.
17. Brown SI, Tragakis MP, Pearce DB: Treatment of the alkali-burned cornea. Am J Ophthalmol 74:316–320, 1972.
18. Slansky HH, Dohlman CH: Collagenase and the cornea. Surv Ophthalmol 14:402–416, 1970.
19. François J, Cambie E, Feher J, Van Den Eeckhout E: Collagenase inhibitors (penicillamine). Ann Ophthalmol 5:391–408, 1973.
20. Pfister RR, Paterson CA: Ascorbic acid in the treatment of alkali burns of the eye. Ophthalmol 87:1050–1057, 1980.
21. Stein MR, Naidoff MA, Dawson CR: Intraocular pressure response to experimental alkali burns. Am J Ophthalmol 75:99–109, 1973.

22. Paterson CA, Pfister RR, Levinson RA: Aqueous humor pH changes after experimental alkali burns. Am J Ophthalmol 79:414–419, 1975.
23. Thoft RA: Conjunctival transplantation as an alternative to keratoplasty. Ophthalmol 86:1084–1092, 1979.
24. Ballen PH, Meltzer M: Lamellar keratoplasty for alkali burns. In *The Cornea: World Congress*. King JH Jr, McTigue JW, eds; London, Butterworth & Co, 1965, 316–324.
25. MacCarthy CF, Hollenhorst RW: Protective moist-chamber eye dressing. Am J Ophthalmol 71:1333–1334, 1971.
26. Callahan A: *Reconstructive Surgery of the Eyelids and Ocular Adnexa*. Birmingham, Ala, Aesculapium Publishing Co, 1966.
27. Hughes WL: *Ophthalmic Plastic Surgery: A Manual Prepared for the Use of Graduates in Medicine*. (Second Edition). Rochester, Minn, American Academy of Ophthalmology and Otolaryngology, 1964.
28. Paton D, Maumenee AE: Surgical management of exposure. In *Plastic and Reconstructive Surgery of the Eye and Adnexa*. Troutman RC, Converse JM, Smith B, eds; London, Butterworth & Co, 1962.
29. Paton D, Milauskas AT: Indications, surgical technique, and results of thin conjunctival flaps on the cornea: a review of 122 consecutive cases. Int Ophthalmol Clin 10:329–345, 1970.
30. Leahey BD: Thermal burns of the eye and adnexa. Am J Ophthalmol 35:1077–1088, 1952.
31. Castroviejo R: The electrokeratome or electromucotome. In *Ophthalmic Plastic Surgery: A Manual Prepared for Use of Graduates in Medicine*. (Second Edition). Hughes WL, ed; Rochester, Minn, American Academy of Ophthalmology and Otolaryngology, 1964, 273–275.
32. Paton D: Pterygium management based upon a theory of pathogenesis. Trans Am Acad Ophthalmol Otolaryngol, 79:603–612, 1975.
33. Cogan DG: Lesions of the eye from radiant energy. JAMA 142:145–151, 1950.
34. Newell FW: Radiant energy and the eye. In *Industrial and Traumatic Ophthalmology: Symposium of the New Orleans Academy of Ophthalmology*. St. Louis, C. V. Mosby Co, 1964, 158–187.
35. Fraunfelder FT, Hanna C: Electric cataracts: I. Sequential changes, unusual and prognostic findings. Arch Ophthalmol 87:179–183, 1972.
36. Duane TD: Valsalva hemorrhagic retinopathy. Am J Ophthalmol 75:637–642, 1973.
37. Zagora E: *Eye Injuries*. Springfield, Ill, Charles C Thomas Co, 1970.
38. Ewald RA, Ritchey CL: Sun gazing as the cause of foveomacular retinitis. Am J Ophthalmol 70:491–497, 1970.
39. Goldberg MF, Young RSL, Read J, Cunha-vaz JG: Macular hole caused by a 589-nanometer dye laser operating for 10 nanoseconds. Retina 3:40–44, 1983.

6

Radiographic and Ultrasonic Imaging in Ocular Injuries

The rapidly changing field of diagnostic imaging has dramatically altered the management of ocular injuries. Time-consuming and inaccurate techniques involving plain tomograms or triangulation have been replaced by rapid, accurate radiographic and ultrasonic scanners. This chapter provides an overview of available techniques that help the treating physician prepare a logical and efficient plan for the workup of the trauma patient.

6.1 HISTORICAL ASPECTS

Diagnosis and localization of ocular and orbital foreign bodies are common indicators for radiologic evaluation. Until recent years, the two most commonly used techniques were the Comberg contact lens and the Sweet external localizer (Figures 6–1 and 6–2). The primary disadvantage of the contact lens is that the eye has been lacerated in the majority of cases in which it is required. The manipulation involved in using it increases the chances for further injury and infection as a result of applying the apparatus directly to the eye. The technique of Sweet involves triangulation using radiopaque markers placed a known distance in front of the eye. Both of these techniques require the key assumption that the eye is of standard dimensions.

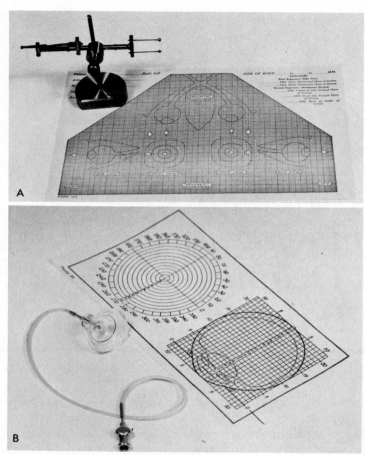

Figure 6–1. Localization devices. (A) Equipment used in Sweet's technique of radiological localization of an intraocular foreign body. (B) Comberg type of corneoscleral lens. The radiopaque ring within the lens is used for localization of an intraocular foreign body.

6.2 TRADITIONAL TECHNIQUES

a. Plain Radiography

The proliferation of sophisticated CT scanners into even small community hospitals has caused many physicians to overlook more routine x-ray studies because of the perception that they are "not as good" as computerized scans. However, in many routine cases a standard radiographic study may yield enough information so that a CT scan is unnecessary. Additionally, there will be occasions where patients may be unable to cooperate for the more lengthy scanning procedure. In such instances, routine radiographs are indispensable.

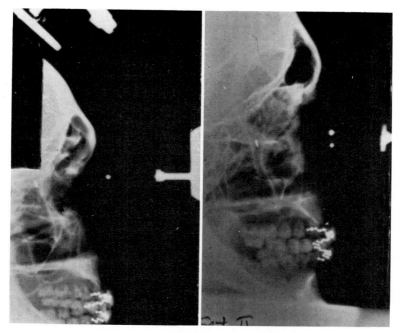

Figure 6–2. Lateral roentgenograms of intraorbital foreign body made with Sweet's apparatus.

b. Soft Tissue Injuries

Soft tissue injuries of the orbit and globe infrequently require plain radiographic evaluation for proper therapy. Lacerations of the lid often are suspected of containing foreign material, which can be demonstrated with either plain film views of the face or bone-free views. Such studies are especially helpful if multiple particles such as buckshot or shattered glass are involved (Figure 6–3).

Injuries involving the extraocular muscles are not usually seen by routine radiographs. They can, as in the case of an orbital floor fracture, be demonstrated indirectly by means of orbitography and tomography (Figure 6–4). CT scanning, however, is the best way to image the muscles. Trauma directly affecting the wall of the eye and the optic nerve is usually not an indication for plain radiographic evaluation except when a foreign body is suspected. Again, CT scanning is the most accurate technique.

c. Orbital Bones

Blunt facial trauma may cause fractures of any of the bones comprising the orbit as well as the optic canal. A variety of specialized views are available, and these views, in conjunction with polytomography, can

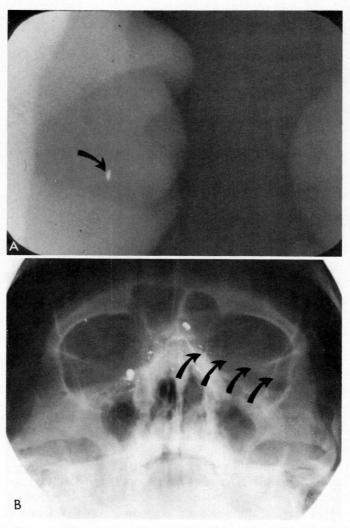

Figure 6–3. The value of lateral bone-free views of the anterior segment of the eye and adnexa. (A) Note silhouette of upper lid, cornea, and lower lid. The radiopaque foreign body (arrow) was not visualized on conventional orbital x-rays. (B) and (C) Posteroanterior and lateral views of another patient who received a shotgun blast to his eye. These routine views suggest multiple intraocular foreign bodies (arrows).

Illustration continued on opposite page

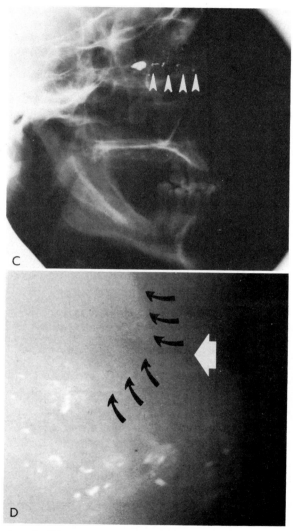

Figure 6–3. *(Continued).* (D) Lateral bone-free view shows multiple foreign bodies superimposed over silhouette of globe (small arrows indicate cornea). Large arrow shows palpebral fissure.

Illustration continued on following page

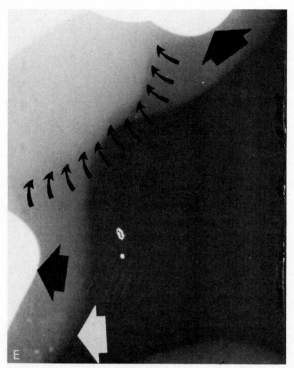

Figure 6–3. *(Continued).* (E) The lateral bone-free view has been repeated with lids withdrawn by Desmarres retractors (large black arrows). The curvature of the cornea is shown by small arrows. All the foreign bodies were in the lower lid (white arrow); none was in the eye.

demonstrate better than 90 per cent of all orbital fractures. Clinical examination should direct the radiologic workup. For example, the study of choice in a patient with orbital emphysema is a Caldwell view, which is excellent for demonstrating medial wall fractures. Table 6–1 provides a list of special views intended to study the various orbital bones.

Polytomography remains an important tool in the evaluation of the bones of the orbit. Although some radiologists now believe that CT scanning is more accurate for diagnosing bony pathology, the majority of radiologists continue to rely on polytomograms. This is an excellent example of an indication for conferral between the ophthalmologist and radiologist prior to ordering imaging studies.

6.3 COMPUTERIZED TOMOGRAPHY
The ability of the CT scanner to study tissues of varying density has made it an invaluable tool for the ophthalmologist, particularly in the setting of

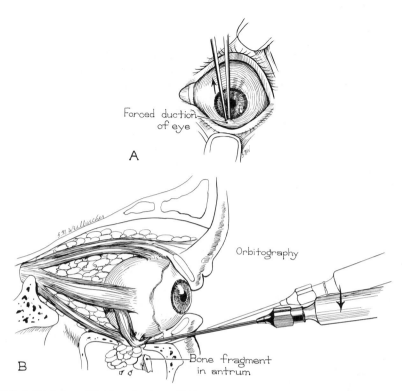

Figure 6–4. Tests for orbital floor fracture. (A) The forced-duction test. Under topical anesthesia the limbal conjunctiva and Tenon's fascia are firmly grasped with a toothed forceps and are tugged superiorly. Resistance to this supraduction is often encountered when orbital tissue is incarcerated in a blow-out fracture of the orbital floor. (B) When the presence of an orbital floor fracture cannot be confirmed by plain x-rays, injection of contrast material is frequently helpful. In order to avoid either perforation of the globe or injection into the muscle cone, the needle should be introduced in the directions shown in the diagram. This orbitographic technique is no longer widely used owing to the availability of technically excellent polytomograms. If polytomography is unavailable or unreliable, the ophthalmologist should personally perform an orbitogram if he is attempting to diagnose a blow-out fracture.

ocular trauma. As with plain x-rays, there are a variety of CT studies available, and the nature of the suspected injury should dictate which study or studies are chosen. A routine CT scan will usually consist of multiple axial or transverse "cuts" beginning at the vertex of the skull and brain and terminating at the level of the base of the skull. The orbital walls, globe, and extraocular muscles are sectioned longitudinally in the horizontal plane. Coronal and sagittal sections are useful for orbital and extraocular examinations.

CT studies can be further enhanced by varying the separation between

Table 6–1. SUGGESTIONS CONCERNING RADIOGRAPHIC PROJECTIONS FOR ORBITAL INJURIES*

Anatomical Site	Optimal Radiographic Projection	Additional Studies
Orbital roof Superior orbital rim	Caldwell (15° PA)	Tomography: particularly suitable to show isolated fractures of the orbital plate or damage of cribriform plate (preferably pluridirectional)
Medial wall		
upper half	Caldwell	Hypocycloidal polytomography
lower half	Special view I (Fueger)**	
Orbital floor		
en face	Waters	Hypocycloidal polytomography
profile	Special view I (Fueger)** Special view II (Fueger)†	Orbitography‡
Lateral wall	Caldwell Rheese Special view II (Fueger)†	Usually not necessary
Infraorbital rim	Waters	Usually not helpful
Optic foramen	Rheese	Tomography (preferably pluridirectional)

Source: From Paton D, Emery J: Injuries of the eye, lids, and the orbit. In *The Management of Trauma*. (Second Edition). Ballinger WF, Rutherford RB, Zuidema GD, eds; Philadelphia, WB Saunders Co, 1973, 219–254. For further information, see Fukado Y: Diagnosis and surgical correction of optic canal fracture after head injury. Ophthalmologica (additamentum) *158*:307–314, 1969; and Milauskas AT, Fueger GF, Schulze RR: Clinical experiences with orbitography in the diagnosis of orbital floor fractures. Trans Am Acad Ophthalmol Otolaryngol *70*:25–39, 1966.

*A facial bone survey should always be obtained to determine the extent of facial trauma. A lateral projection should be included to show the facial bones in a second plane. Special projections with narrow collimation should follow the facial bone survey. Technical excellence is necessary. There must be no motion. The density range should be long.

**Fueger I. Forehead-film position, C/R 30 degrees caudad, to exit 1 to 1¼ inches below nasion.

†Fueger II. Oblique position, sagittal plane rotated 20 degrees, C/R 35 degrees caudad, through affected orbit, to exit 1 inch below infraorbital rim.

‡Extraconal orbitography can be performed to demonstrate defects in the lower medial orbital wall and in the orbital floor. The procedure consists of scout radiographs, anesthesia of the lower lid, injection of contrast material into the extraconal fatty tissue space along the orbital floor, and postinjection radiographs. Local anesthetic: 2% lidocaine (Xylocaine). Contrast material: mixture of 3.5 ml of 50% diatrizoate sodium (Hypaque), 3 ml of 2% lidocaine, 0.5 ml of diluent containing 150 units of hyaluronidase (Wydase), prepared fresh prior to use. Approximately 6 ml of the mixture is injected through a No. 22 needle 1½ inches long. The series of radiographs consists of Special view I, Special view II, Waters, and Lateral, taken before and immediately after injection. (For further information, see Fueger GF, Milauskas AT, Britton W: The roentgenologic evaluation of orbital blow-out injuries. Am J Roentgenol Radium Ther Nucl Med *97*:614–617, 1966.)

cuts, but unless otherwise specified an 8-mm separation is used for most studies. The most currently available scanners are capable of 2-mm cuts, although the most recent "state of the art" instruments are capable of 1-mm or thinner cuts. With increased scanner speed, the length of these more detailed studies is only slightly prolonged over that of routine x-ray studies. Radiopaque contrast media may be infused during the scan to demonstrate vascularized lesions but are not usually necessary when evaluating ocular injuries. Table 6–2 summarizes some of the indications for the use of CT scanning in a setting of ocular trauma.

a. Soft Tissue Injuries

CT scanning has supplanted plain x-rays in many indications of ocular soft tissue injuries and in certain instances may be ordered in lieu of routine films. Scanner orientation is determined by the nature of the injury; e.g., a knife injury suspected of having transected the optic nerve is an indication for an axial scan with 2-mm cuts through the posterior orbit. A blow-out fracture with possible muscle incarceration is best demonstrated with coronal sections through the orbital floor and maxillary antrum.

b. Orbital Fractures

The resolving power of current CT scanners is approaching a level at which only subtle fractures of the orbital walls will not be detected. The

Table 6–2. POSSIBLE CT SCAN DIAGNOSES

I. Extraocular soft tissue damage
   A. Hematoma
      1. Lids
      2. Extraocular muscles
      3. Orbit
      4. Optic nerve sheath
   B. Direct tissue damage
      1. Transected muscle
      2. Incarcerated muscle
      3. Transected optic nerve
   C. Ocular and intraocular damage
      1. Dislocated lens
      2. Vitreous hemorrhage
      3. Choroidal detachment
      4. Retinal detachment
      5. Ruptured globe
      6. Foreign body (globe or orbit)
II. Orbital bones
   A. Blow-out fracture
   B. Fractures of optic canal
   C. Secondary sinus involvement

location and extent of the fracture can usually be demonstrated. In addition, it can be used to determine which soft tissues are incarcerated in the fracture. In blow-out fractures of the orbital floor it is possible to demonstrate that either fat alone or fat and inferior rectus muscle are incarcerated. There may be some predictive value as to whether or not surgical repair is indicated based on these findings.[1]

c. Foreign Bodies of the Eye and Orbit

There is as yet no single imaging device that can determine the presence and exact location of an ocular foreign body in all instances. The physician must therefore intelligently choose and utilize a variety of imaging techniques. As emphasized in Chapter 4, the most valuable technique for intraocular foreign body localization is direct examination with the ophthalmoscope. Every attempt should be made to complete a thorough ophthalmoscopic examination prior to sending the patient for lengthy radiologic evaluation.

CT scanning now enables the ocular trauma surgeon to locate foreign bodies with relative precision despite opaque media (see Figure 4–18). The physician should order both axial and coronal sections with 1- to 2-mm cuts through the orbit. This scanning technique will detect foreign bodies smaller than 1 mm of varying composition and density. The exact location of the foreign body may be accurately determined in a majority of cases, and copies of the scans should be available in the operating room to help guide surgical removal. It may be difficult to determine the exact location of small metallic foreign bodies lying near or within the sclera because of the artifacts they cause. Occasionally it is impossible to determine whether the foreign body is actually in the globe. The radiologist may vary the CT "window" to reduce such artifacts and make localization more accurate. Direct communication with the radiologist performing the scan is essential in this instance.

d. Timing of Vitrectomy

The proper timing of vitrectomy to remove opacities in the ocular media following primary closure of penetrating ocular injuries remains a challenge. In many cases, sustained hypotony prior to and during the repair results in ciliary body and choroidal detachments.[2] In other cases, suprachoroidal hemorrhage clears very slowly. In such instances, pars plana incisions for the vitrectomy instruments are hazardous. CT scans can often demonstrate these defects, and sequential use of this technique can be used to follow their disappearance. As the uvea becomes reattached, the physician can prepare the patient for surgery.

6.4 ULTRASOUND

Recent years have seen an increase in both the accuracy and availability of ocular ultrasonic scanners. When CT scanning is unavailable, ultrasound can provide much of the same information. Specifically, intraocular and orbital foreign bodies can often be identified and localized. Ultrasound has the advantage of being a dynamic examination with which an almost infinite number of views may be obtained including studies of the moving globe. Additionally, most ultrasound units are portable and may be brought to the bedside of patients otherwise too ill to move or to the operating room for examinations under sterile surgical conditions.

The principal disadvantage of ultrasound is that direct contact with the lid or globe is necessary. As many patients undergoing ultrasonic examination will be suspected of having open globes, care must be taken to maintain sterility and avoid unnecessary pressure on the eye. The probe may be kept sterile by ensheathing it in a surgical glove.

a. Foreign Bodies

Ultrasound will only rarely be able to determine the presence of a foreign body where CT scanning and plain x-rays have failed. Ultrasound, however, may be helpful in localizing foreign bodies within the eye when they are located near the ocular wall. This is a case in which the artifacts from a foreign body imaged with the CT scanner may interfere with the radiologist's ability to tell whether the foreign body is within the wall of the eye or just outside of the globe.

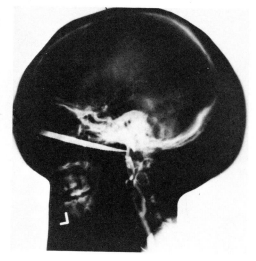

Figure 6–5. Angiogram of patient in Figure 4–23. After examining the entire study, the tip of the knife was determined to be approximately 10 mm from the middle meningeal artery.

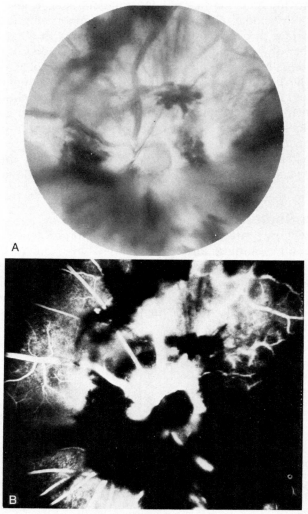

Figure 6–6. Optic nerve avulsion following injury with a basketball. (A) Hemorrhage surrounds the nerve head. (B) The fluorescein angiogram on the day of injury reveals persistent filling of the retinal circulation.

b. Diagnosis of Intraocular Pathology

Ultrasound is most helpful in the diagnosis of retinal detachment, choroidal detachment, and intravitreal hemorrhage. These conditions must be detected and completely evaluated prior to commencing operative intervention, as they will alter the surgical approach. As mentioned previously, ultrasound may be used under the sterile conditions of the operating room.

6.5 ANGIOGRAPHY

a. Arteriography and Venography

Carotid arteriography and head and neck venography must sometimes be used in the evaluation of injuries involving the eye and orbit. This is especially true when a missile injury is involved. The arteriogram helps to identify the location of any foreign bodies with respect to major blood vessels. In addition, however, it is often critically important to rule out any damage to vital vessels. The finding of excessive bleeding or a large hematoma in the face or neck makes consultation with a head and neck or vascular surgeon mandatory. These consultants will then help in the planning of proper imaging techniques.

When the surgeon contemplates removal of a foreign body, it is sometimes necessary to determine whether major vessels are likely to be encountered during the operation. This is vividly demonstrated in Figure 6–5.

b. Fluorescein Angiography

Fluorescein angiography is sometimes useful in demonstrating vascular sequelae of trauma. Avulsion of the optic nerve has been demonstrated to occur with preservation of part of the retinal vasculature[3] (Figure 6–6). In addition, foreign bodies may sever vessels, resulting in branch arterial occlusions.

References

1. Gilbard SM, Mafee MF, Lagouros PA, Langer BG: The prognostic significance of computed tomography of orbital blowout fractures. (In press)
2. Peyman GA, Mafee M, Schulman J: Computed tomography in choroidal detachment. Ophthalmology 91:156–162, 1984.
3. Chow AY, Goldberg MF, Frenkel M: Evulsion of the optic nerve in association with basketball injuries. Ann Ophthalmol 16:35–37, 1984.

Abrasions of the Globe

7.1 TECHNIQUES OF EXAMINATION

a. Lid Eversion

Corneal abrasions are often due to foreign bodies caught under the upper lid, and every physician should know how to evert the lid. There will be many opportunities to remove what are colloquially referred to as "cinders" or "trash" from the inner aspects of the lids (see Figure 4–4).

The patient is seated and asked to look down; the upper lid, grasped by its central lashes, is pulled downward and slightly outward; the examiner then presses with a finger, cotton applicator, or other blunt instrument at the upper margin of the tarsus and maintains this gentle pressure while the lid is flipped into an everted position. Maintenance of downward gaze is essential as it relaxes the levator muscle, and the examiner should constantly remind the patient to continue looking down. A drop of topical anesthetic should be used if the patient is too uncomfortable to permit full cooperation. For return to normal lid position, the patient is directed to look up, and the pull of the levator muscle will usually restore the normal anatomic relationship. A gentle pull on the lashes in an outward and downward direction will help flip the tarsus into normal position.

Double eversion of the lid is sometimes necessary to inspect the otherwise inaccessible superior conjunctival fornix. The lid is first singly everted, and a Desmarres retractor is then placed between the two skin surfaces with the retractor portion engaging the tarsus (see Figure 4–5). Gentle upward and outward traction will then expose the fornix. Excessive force should be avoided, as it can result in disinsertion of the levator muscle.

b. Instruments of Illumination

The most obvious source of illumination is a pocket penlight. When fully charged, this will project a bright and relatively well-focused beam of light if held close to the object of regard. Another easily found illuminator is known as a transilluminator or "Finhoff" light. This casts a bright and highly focused beam of light from several inches away. Versions of this light that fit onto standard ophthalmoscope handles are manufactured and should be available in an emergency room where eye patients are regularly examined (see Figure 1–1).

Many emergency rooms are outfitted with slit lamps, and this instrument is a mainstay of ophthalmic examination. The combination of a focused and variably shaped light beam and biomicroscopic magnification gives the skilled practitioner a great advantage in diagnosing and treating subtle abrasions of the globe.

c. Fluorescein

This hydrophilic dye is used to detect and outline the extent of epithelial defects. Because it is repelled by the lipid cell membranes of the epithelial cells, it only stains areas in which the epithelium is missing, and the fluorescein has access to the high water content of the underlying stroma.

Sterile, fluorescein-impregnated paper strips are readily available, and single-use dropperettes of highly concentrated solutions may also be used. Aqueous solutions of fluorescein do not readily maintain sterility, and they afford an excellent culture medium for *Pseudomonas.* Therefore, the dropperettes should be discarded after one use.

7.2 COMMON ABRASION SYNDROMES

There is hardly a person who has not known the anguish of a corneal abrasion. Upon injury, there is sudden onset of pain, lacrimation, and blepharospasm. Blinking and motions of the eyeball aggravate the pain. Even in the absence of an actual foreign body, a foreign-body sensation is produced no matter how small the abrasion might be. Such eyes are not easily examined until afforded immediate relief by a drop of topical anesthetic (not ointment) such as tetracaine 1% or proparacaine hydrochloride 0.5%.

a. Scratches

Although an intact blink reflex is usually sufficient to prevent corneal damage, any one of a number of guided missiles can penetrate the normal defenses. Common among them are fingernails, sand and dirt blowing in the air, hairbrushes, mascara wands, and misdirected eyelashes. A careful history must always be pursued, as it will direct the search for occult foreign bodies and perforations and may alert the physician to the possible contamination of the abraded cornea with pathogenic organisms.

b. Contact Lenses

Contact lenses are the most common foreign bodies found in the cornea, and, with millions of them in use, the frequency of minor problems associated with them is not surprising. There are three major reasons for acute discomfort caused by contact lenses: a foreign body between the lens and cornea; improper fit (or a defective lens); and damage to the corneal epithelium on insertion or removal of the lens. In each case, abrasion or edema of corneal epithelium is the cause for discomfort, which is precisely the same in character as that resulting from other foreign bodies and abrasions.

Removal of a contact lens under conditions of pain, lacrimation, and photophobia can be quite difficult and requires patience. Find a comfortable place for the patient to sit where there is enough light to visualize the position of the lens. Instillation of a drop of topical anesthetic is very helpful. The lens is removed from the cornea by sliding it to the inferior portion of the bulbar conjunctiva as follows: place an index finger on the lens and ask the patient to look up; this will slide the lens onto the inferior bulbar conjunctiva; while reminding the patient to maintain an upward gaze, either grasp the lens between the thumb and index finger (in the case of a soft lens) or use the margin of the upper lid to elevate the superior pole of the lens off of the eye and break the suction that holds it against the globe (in the case of a hard lens). In either case the lens is now held between the thumb and index finger and placed into a solution of sterile saline.

Fluorescein staining of the cornea after removal of the contact lens is helpful in determining the cause of the abrasion. A diffuse central area of mild fluorescein staining and edema suggests that the lens has been worn too long or is too "tight." Small irregular abrasions (usually on the inferior cornea near the limbus) are probably related to difficulties in inserting or removing the lens. Irregular linear scratches of the corneal epithelium are characteristic of changes found when there has been a foreign body between the contact lens and the cornea. It is helpful to examine the lens under high-power magnification to see if there are defective edges, cracks, or foreign bodies on the posterior surface of the lens.

Management of the eye abraded by a contact lens is the same as that for other forms of corneal abrasions. It is wise to delay restarting contact lens wear until two days after the symptoms have resolved.

One word of caution should be sounded. An increase in the number of bacterial corneal ulcers has occurred with the increased use of contact lenses, particularly extended-wear soft lenses. Ocular irritation in these patients should never be passed off as "overwear" without an examination of the cornea to rule out the presence of a suppurative process.

c. Sunlamp-induced Corneal Abrasion

As the drive in our society to maintain year-round suntans has escalated, the incidence of ultraviolet burns of the cornea has risen along with the sales of sunlamps. Another cause of the same syndrome is the use of a welding or carbon arc without proper eye protection. There is typically an interval of six to ten hours after exposure before symptoms appear; thereafter, the patient notes an irritated, foreign-body sensation of the eyes that progresses to severe photophobia, pain, and blepharospasm. Examination shows mild chemosis, and topically applied fluorescein produces a punctate staining of the cornea.

d. Recurrent Erosion

Small linear scratches of the cornea from a sharp object such as an infant's fingernail or a piece of paper can lead to recurrent healing problems rarely found with blunt abrasion.[1] The pathogenesis of recurrent erosion appears related to damage to the basement membrane of the epithelium.[2] Acute pain may recur days, weeks, or even months after the original injury, since the basement membrane does not become totally remodeled for up to three months after it has been disrupted. The patient is often awakened from sleep early in the morning with a foreign-body sensation. This probably occurs because the epithelial cells become hypoxic and edematous during sleep and, when swollen, are easily lifted from the underlying abnormal basement membrane. A flap of detached epithelium is often seen overlying the original site of abrasion.

Wearing a semi-pressure patch for 24 hours and applying a hyperosmotic ointment (sodium chloride solution, 5%) at bedtime for several weeks will often arrest the distressing series of acute and painful episodes. The therapeutic use of a soft contact lens may provide successful management when simpler means have failed. Ultimately, debridement of the entire corneal epithelium is sometimes necessary to allow the epithelial basement membrane to "start from scratch."

e. Herpetic Keratitis

A foreign-body sensation in the eye may be the first manifestation of herpes simplex keratitis. Not only can the discomfort of this common ocular infection simulate a foreign body in the conjunctival sac, but this viral infection may follow corneal trauma by allowing the virus entrance to the cornea at the site of epithelial damage. Fluorescein staining of the cornea may reveal a characteristic dendritic pattern, but this is not a consistent enough finding to rely on. Herpetic infections are characteristically associated with decreased or absent corneal sensation, although this is difficult to test for in a recently injured eye.

It is well known that steroids are contraindicated for superficial herpetic infections of the cornea; therefore, since it is difficult to differentiate between herpetic infection and minimal corneal trauma and since an injured cornea is prone to viral infection, *no medication containing a steroid should ever be used in eyes with a corneal abrasion.*

f. Corneal Foreign Bodies

Foreign bodies lodged on the surface of the cornea can be single or multiple, grossly visible or scarcely detected on slit-lamp examination. Wind-blown grit, fragments of insects, fragments of glass, thorns, caterpillar hairs, and similar splinter-shaped objects are representative invaders, although almost any physical or biologic object may be found. Most of these particles remain superficial and can be readily removed with a saline-moistened cotton swab after a drop of topical anesthetic is placed on the eye.

Metallic foreign bodies are commonly found in on-the-job ocular accidents. Rust is often deposited on the cornea while the patient lies under the body of a car; small pieces of metal may elude the barrier of the eyelids while the patient operates a grinding wheel; a piece of hammer may fly off and hit the cornea while the patient pounds on a piece of metal or concrete.

If the patient waits a day or two for treatment, a rust ring may surround the foreign body. The patient is brought to the slit lamp and after topical anesthetic has been applied, the metal fragment is lifted from the crater in which it sits with a 25-gauge needle on a syringe (Figure 7–1). A saline-moistened cotton applicator is then touched to the piece of

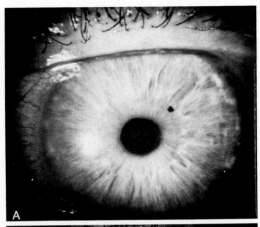

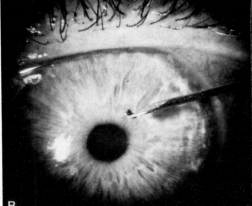

Figure 7–1. Steps in removal of a corneal foreign body. (A) While the eyelids are retracted, the foreign body is viewed at the slit lamp with diffuse illumination. (B) A small needle is used to lift the foreign body out of the crater in the cornea in which it lays. (C) A moistened cotton-tipped applicator is touched to the foreign body, which clings to it and is lifted away from the eye. (From Deutsch TA, Feller DB: Injuries of the eye, the lids and the orbit. In *The Management of Trauma* (Fourth Edition). Zuidema GD, et al, eds; Philadelphia, WB Saunders Co, 1985.)

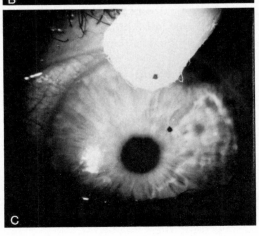

metal to remove it from the cornea. Rust rings may be removed either at the time of the first examination or several days later when they often can easily be lifted from the cornea as a firm cast. A dental burr, when available, is a safe tool to remove rust rings.

Explosions sometimes drive multiple foreign bodies into the corneal epithelium (see Figure 4–2). In such cases, additional scarring can occur from attempts to curette each particle individually. Thus, at least as the first portion of the procedure, denuding the entire epithelium with an alcohol- or ether-soaked cotton-tipped applicator is indicated. Bowman's membrane will be spared, and all the superficial foreign bodies will be easily removed, leaving only those few that are deeper for more vigorous extraction techniques. The epithelial defect will be covered within several days. Deep corneal foreign bodies that are not inciting a reaction in the cornea or anterior chamber usually should be left in place.

Occasionally, a deep foreign body must be removed because it is causing a keratitis or iritis or because it has or is threatening to enter the anterior chamber. An operating microscope should be used to optimize the patient's comfort and the physician's view of the operative field. If entrance into the eye is a possibility, the patient should be prepped and draped as for all intraocular surgery.

In most cases, a corneal foreign body should be removed along the path of its entrance, whether perpendicular or tangential to the surface of the cornea. The latter situation is the more difficult. With a fine needle introduced into the tract at the site of entry, it is often possible to tease a foreign body such as glass or wood back through its entry path. Fibrillar material, in particular, is more completely removed by this technique than by performing a separate "cut down" perpendicular to the location of the foreign body. Such surgery increases the area of corneal damage and requires a much bigger incision in the corneal stroma.

7.3 TREATMENT OF CORNEAL DEFECTS

Any disruption of the corneal epithelium may result in a reflexive break-down of the blood-aqueous barrier. The result is a low-grade iridocyclitis. In this situation, the patient will be much more comfortable if a short- or medium-acting cycloplegic (cyclopentolate hydrochloride, 1%, or homa-tropine, 5%) is instilled in the eye prior to the placement of a patch.

A broad-spectrum antibiotic ointment (gentamicin, tobramycin, or Neosporin) is customarily placed in the eye. Although ointments retard corneal epithelial healing in the experimental situation, in practice they do not appear to adversely affect the resolution of most abrasions. The clinical need for an antibiotic has not been demonstrated, and many practitioners omit this portion of the therapy.

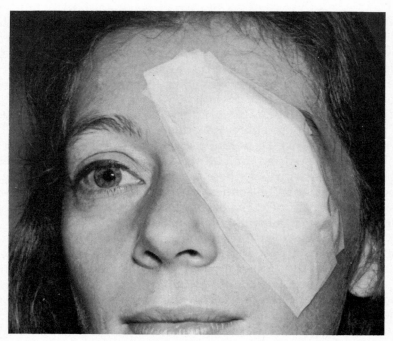

Figure 7–2. A semipressure eye dressing affords comfort and protection when properly applied. The lids are closed under the patch. The tape is placed to avoid impairment of the ipsilateral side of the face and should be lateral to the nasolabial fold to prevent inconvenience with eating and talking. Note that no tape crosses the nose.

A semi-pressure patch (Figure 7–2) is placed on the eye as follows: with the eyes gently closed, an eye pad is folded in half and placed on the eyelid; a second patch is placed horizontally over the first and is held in place with the thumb and index finger; tape is placed over the pads so that the pieces run from the center of the forehead to the malar eminence. The patch is taped tightly enough so that the lid cannot be opened. The oblique orientation of the tape prevents it from loosening when the patient moves the jaw to eat or speak.

Topical anesthetics must never be given to the patient to take home, as they retard wound healing, aggravate the keratitis, and become a virtual addiction for pain relief.[3] We treat several patients with corneal ulcers each year referred to us by nonophthalmologists who have treated the patients with topical anesthetics. In addition, it is worth repeating the warning that topical steroid preparations have no place in the treatment of traumatic corneal abrasions, and they should be scrupulously avoided.

Most small corneal abrasions will heal in 24 to 48 hours. The patient should leave the patch in place for that period and return for follow-up care in one or two days. Mild analgesics are occasionally necessary, especially in cases of linear abrasions such as fingernail injuries. Sleeping seems to aid epithelial healing, and many patients who have been kept awake all night by a painful abrasion will be so relieved by the patch that they return after a good night's sleep with the epithelial surface restored.

Since the predisposition for a corneal ulcer remains until the epithelium has completely healed, no patient should be discharged from care until that time. Once the abrasion has healed, a complete eye exam should be performed to rule out any other pathology that may have been inflicted during the original injury.

References

1. Thygeson P: Observations of recurrent erosion of the cornea. Am J Ophthalmol 47(no. 5, pt. 2):48–51, 1959.
2. Khodadoust AA, Silverstein AM, Kenyon KR, Dowling JE: Adhesion of regenerating corneal epithelium: the role of basement membrane. Am J Ophthalmol 65:339–348, 1968.
3. Epstein DL, Paton D: Keratitis from misuse of corneal anesthetics. N Engl J Med 279:396–399, 1968.

CHAPTER

8

Lacerations of the Globe

8.1 PRELIMINARY CONSIDERATIONS

From the time that the ophthalmologist realizes that an injured eye will require surgery, the plan for surgical repair should be formulated in sequential steps. This must be a carefully considered approach, but one that is subject to immediate change, depending on the events and findings during the preoperative evaluation and surgery. Moreover, the plan must be formulated in advance to be certain that the proper instruments are available and to allow the repair to proceed with the greatest efficiency and safety for the injured eye.

The less experienced surgeon should take the time to jot down the anticipated steps of the forthcoming operation and should make a drawing of the damaged eye, indicating the location of anticipated stab incisions, full limbal incisions, diathermy or cryotherapy sites, and so forth. Complications such as uveal bleeding, vitreous loss, or difficulty with closing the wound or restoring the anterior chamber must be anticipated and their management considered.

8.2 REPAIR VERSUS ENUCLEATION

No matter how severe a penetrating ocular injury is, primary repair should almost invariably be attempted. Increasingly, salvage is accomplished in

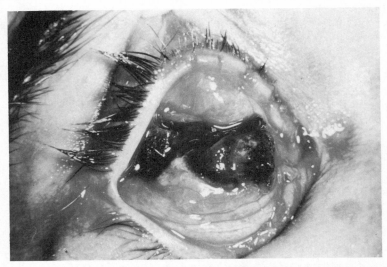

Figure 8–1. A grinding-wheel fragment struck this patient's eye, causing total destruction of the globe, retention of large pieces of stone, and loss of light perception. In this case, after photography and informed consent, a primary enucleation was performed because there was no possibility of salvaging the eye.

the face of seemingly overwhelming odds. Furthermore, the patient appreciates the fact that maximum effort was made. Enucleation can always be carried out soon enough to avoid sympathetic ophthalmia if the postoperative eye has no chance of return of useful vision. Primary enucleation is justified only when the globe is totally disorganized (Figure 8–1) or in the face of severe retinal prolapse. In addition, the patient must be alert and sober prior to surgery and must give written informed consent in advance.

8.3 PREOPERATIVE EVALUATION

a. Techniques of Examination

Obviously, a thorough preoperative examination is highly desirable. Patients with post-traumatic lid swelling, deep lid lacerations, or otherwise damaged periocular tissues require examination of the globe itself with a thoroughness inversely proportional to the ease of the examination (Figure 8–2). However, when the eye has been lacerated, pressure on the globe must be avoided assiduously. An upper lid can be retracted by gentle pulling from the superior orbital rim with the thumb. All pressure should be applied to the brow and no pressure to the eyeball itself. If the view is still inadequate, topical anesthetic is instilled (from a new, sterile bottle), and lid retractors are used with notable gentleness.

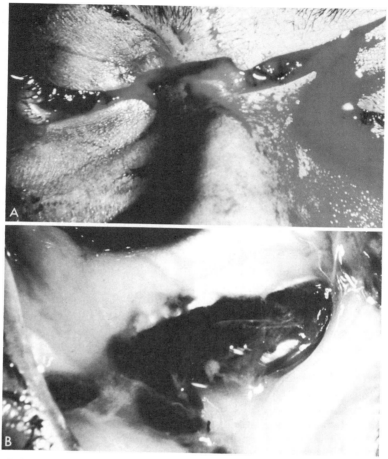

Figure 8–2. (A) This patient was slashed across the eyelids with a knife. (B) The accident room physician, concentrating on the lid lesions, failed to discover that the globe of the right eye was also lacerated, with uveal prolapse.

The surgeon must use individual judgment in determining the extent of preoperative examination in inebriated and uncooperative adults and in infants and children; a struggling patient may make examination of the eye hazardous as well as ineffective. With many helping hands and "mummy wraps," a young child can be held so immobile that struggles cease and cooperation may become remarkably good. Alternatively, completion of the examination may await general anesthesia.

Despite the fact that the surgeon will use an operating microscope, the preliminary slit-lamp examination may provide more precise information than that which can be obtained in the operating room. For example, if a patient has a corneoscleral laceration with blood and fibrin in the anterior chamber, the physician often can more readily determine the presence or absence of lens involvement before the patient reaches the operating room.

b. Hidden and Occult Injuries

The appearance of a corneal or scleral laceration needs little description. However, a scleral rupture or laceration can be hidden under hemorrhagic or edematous conjunctiva and Tenon's fascia, and occasionally the signs of serious intraocular damage are mild. When perforating injuries are more obvious, the anterior chamber is often flat or shallow and may contain blood. The iris or the ciliary body may be incarcerated in the wound or prolapsed through it (Figure 8–3). Similarly, if the eye is quiet but the pupil is markedly peaked, one must suspect a perforation of the sclera. In such a case, the peaked pupil points to the perforation.

Frequently, there is external bleeding from the injured sclera and uvea. Subconjunctival hemorrhage and chemosis seemingly out of proportion to the injury should make one suspicious that a perforation of the sclera lies under the hemorrhage.

It is not always easy to determine whether the lens has been damaged; hemorrhage may obscure the view, and rapid accumulation of fibrin in the pupillary space is sometimes indistinguishable from flocculent lens cortex or vitreous. The entire lens, along with some of the vitreous, can be extruded through the wound, and the lens may be wiped away when the injury is first inspected. If this is the case, such information must be noted on the patient's record in the event that other physicians later assume care of the patient. Rarely, the lens is luxated via a scleral rupture into the subconjunctival space, where it may be unrecognized (Figure 8–4). Patients who have had previous intraocular surgery are likely to have ruptures along the original surgical wound and may have extrusion of intraocular contents through the rupture (Figure 8–5).

Ultrasonograms, conventional x-rays, and computerized tomograms are helpful in determining the status of the vitreous cavity and retina when visualization with an ophthalmoscope is impossible. The use of these modalities is discussed in Chapter 6.

Minor brow and lid lacerations (Figures 8–6 through 8–11) may be associated with scleral and retinal perforation, even when the external lacerations are apparently remote from the globe.[1] Signs of scleral perforation need not be present. This appears to occur most often with injuries caused by narrow, sharp objects such as darts, scissors, or knives. *The necessity of suspecting a perforating injury to the globe in such cases cannot be overemphasized.*

Conjunctival lacerations may be observed underlying a lid puncture and should suggest the possibility of an associated perforation of the

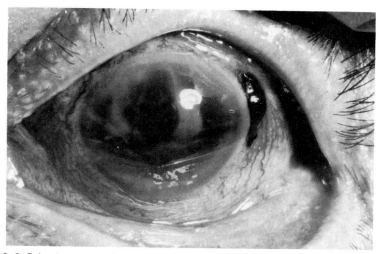

Figure 8–3. Scleral rupture at the limbus after blunt trauma. Iris and ciliary body have prolapsed into the subconjunctival space.

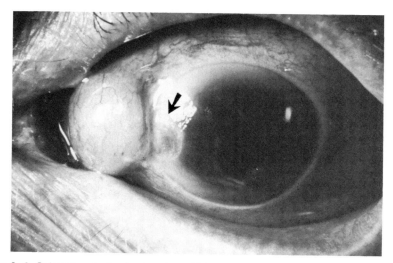

Figure 8–4. Subconjunctival scleral rupture. This rupture (similar to that in Figure 8–3) has also occurred from blunt trauma; however, the lens has luxated through the scleral rupture at the limbus and occupies a position at the limbus, causing such elevation of perilimbal tissue that tear-film inadequacy has led to dellen of the peripheral cornea (arrow).

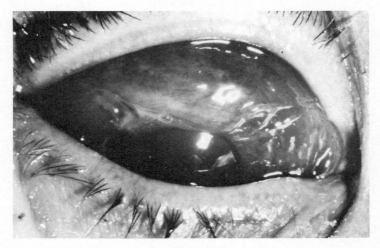

Figure 8–5. Subconjunctival intraocular lens following trauma. An extracapsular cataract extraction and placement of an intraocular lens was performed one year previous because of a cataract secondary to this patient's retinitis pigmentosa. On the day of the injury, the patient bent over and struck her eye on the edge of a chair. On examination, the intraocular lens could be seen prolapsed beneath the conjunctiva. The eye ultimately became phthisical.

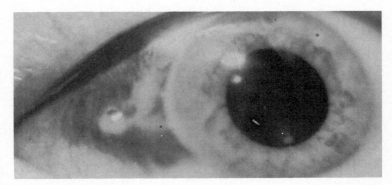

Figure 8–6. A conjunctival hemorrhage signals the location of a perforating injury caused by a wire. The puncture wound was self-sealing. The patient was treated only with antibiotics, and the eye was salvaged.

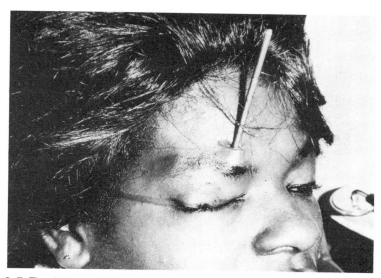

Figure 8–7. The right eye of this 20-year-old victim of an ice-pick attack was undamaged. The pick entered above the brow and passed through lid tissue, exited at the gray line, passed through bulbar conjunctiva, and stopped at the inferior orbital rim. (Photograph reproduced through the courtesy of John L. Barnes, M.D.)

eyeball itself (see Figure 8–8). However, edema and exudate may frequently obscure small (1 to 2 mm) conjunctival lacerations, or, if visible, the lacerations may appear so benign and inconsequential that scleral involvement may not be suspected. *More importantly, an instrument that penetrates the peripheral aspect of the lid or brow may pass into the globe without encountering the conjunctiva at all.*

When sharp, narrow instruments (needles, pins, darts, wires, scissors, ice picks, or knives) perforate the globe, many of the classic signs of scleral perforation, such as lid edema, chemosis, perilimbal hyperemia, lacrimation, persistent hypotony, and vitreous hemorrhage, may be absent. Such small punctures may be sealed by incarcerated uveal tissue or by the sclera itself. Under such circumstances, the scleral and retinal perforations can be termed "occult." Of paramount importance is the consideration that such perforations might exist, even when the lid or brow laceration appears trivial, healed, or remote from the globe. Otherwise, an appreciable delay between initial examination and appropriate therapy may occur. In particular, *the finding of normal, or even elevated, intraocular pressure should never convince the surgeon that a perforation has not occurred.* Small puncture sites are commonly plugged with uvea or vitreous, and lacerations under the insertions of the rectus muscles are notorious for failing to cause hypotony. Even rapidly leaking small corneal

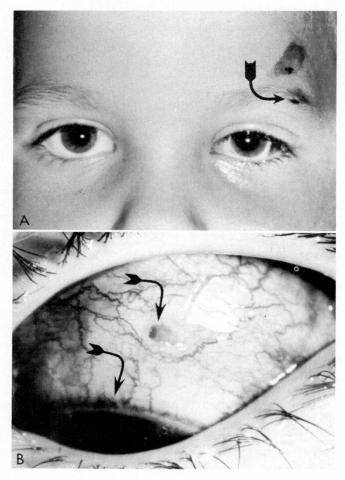

Figure 8–8. This case is similar to that shown in Figure 8–7 but with more serious injury. (A) Brow puncture is indicated by arrow. (B) Underlying occult perforation of globe. The lower arrow indicates the superior limbus; the upper arrow shows scleral puncture, initially overlooked. A clue to the presence of ocular damage is the conjunctival hemorrhage best seen in (A). (Photographs reproduced with the permission of Goldberg MF, Tessler HH: Occult intraocular perforations from brow and lid lacerations. Arch Ophthalmol 86:145–149, 1971.)

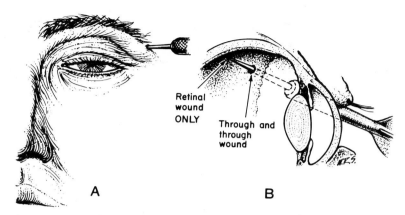

Figure 8–9. (A) Puncture through lateral aspect of brow results in occult damage to globe causing (B) a single scleral but a double retinal perforation. (Drawing reproduced with the permission of Goldberg MF, Tessler HH: Occult intraocular perforations from brow and lid lacerations. Arch Ophthalmol 86:145–149, 1971.)

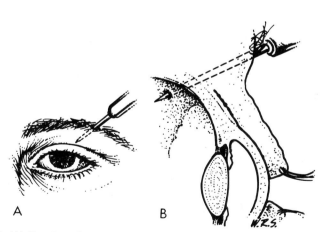

Figure 8–10. (A) Puncture through brow causes (B) occult single perforation of sclera and single perforation of retina. (Drawing reproduced with the permission of Goldberg MF, Tessler HH: Occult intraocular perforations from brow and lid lacerations. Arch Ophthalmol 86:145–149, 1971.)

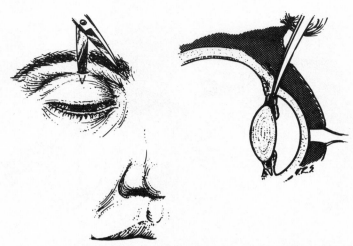

Figure 8–11. Scissors perforating upper lid cause occult scleral and lens damage. (Drawing reproduced with the permission of Goldberg MF, Tessler HH: Occult intraocular perforations from brow and lid lacerations. Arch Ophthalmol 86:145–149, 1971.)

lacerations can be associated with a formed anterior chamber and normal intraocular pressure.

Trauma of this nature may include different types of retinal involvement, such as a single scleral perforation associated with single retinal perforation (see Figure 8–10), double scleral perforation associated with double retinal perforation, a solitary scleral entry site associated with double retinal perforation (see Figure 8–9), or a scleral entry through the ciliary body coupled with involvement of more distant areas of the retina.

Because progressive cataractous changes (see Figure 4–7) and vitreous hemorrhage may rapidly obscure an important retinal lesion, *careful inspection of the retina should be considered an urgent priority when the slightest possibility of scleral perforation exists.* Indirect ophthalmoscopy through a maximally dilated pupil remains the best technique for detecting such retinal involvement. *There is no contraindication to dilatation of the pupil with sterile eyedrops in the face of a known or suspected ocular perforation.* Adequate examination may require general anesthesia, especially in children, in whom injuries with sharp pointed objects are common. If ophthalmoscopy is unsuccessful or incomplete, surgical exploration of the sclera should be considered necessary.

Almost all scleral perforations should be surgically closed. Possible consequences of unrepaired scleral perforation include progressive vitreous loss and retinal herniation, retinal detachment, connective tissue ingrowth, infection, staphyloma formation, continued hemorrhage, and a lengthened healing period. Although it may be argued that many eyes without perforation will be needlessly explored, the severity of these potential complications appears to outweigh the minimal trauma of a conjunctival peritomy and scleral exploration. It is true that certain self-sealing scleral lacerations require no sutures for proper healing. These self-sealing properties cannot, however, be appreciated prior to direct visualization.

Whether or not tiny retinal tears from perforating injuries require prophylactic obliteration (by photocoagulation, scleral diathermy, or scleral cryotherapy with or without scleral buckling) remains uncertain. In comparison, deeply placed scleral sutures may cause peripheral retinal tears at the time of strabismus surgery. In most cases, these relatively atraumatic small scleral and retinal tears heal without subsequent retinal detachment. However, larger wounds, especially when they are jagged, contaminated, and associated with bleeding in the vitreous, may have considerably more serious consequences: vitreous disorganization and fibrosis, infection, and retinal detachment. Consequently, on balance, prophylactic obliteration of an associated retinal tear and closure of a scleral defect appear to have significant merit.[1]

c. Prophylaxis Against Infection

Early during the evaluation of the patient, cultures, which may be helpful in the future if the patient develops an infection, should be obtained. The conjunctiva should be wiped with a culture swab and the conjunctival flora determined. In addition, if the weapon or object that caused the injury is available, it should also be cultured. If the patient develops an infection postoperatively, the preoperative cultures may provide a clue as to what antibiotics are necessary.

Any patient with a penetrating injury should be started on intravenous antibiotics. Although the need for this aggressive treatment has not been demonstrated in a double-masked clinical trial, most series of post-traumatic endophthalmitis include many patients in whom no IV antibiotics were used. In addition, very few patients who are treated with IV antibiotics will develop endophthalmitis. Therefore, until better data are available to resolve this controversy, it seems justifiable to start all such patients on IV therapy.

The use of antibiotics is discussed more fully in Chapter 9. However, the combination of methicillin, penicillin, and gentamicin has proven to be efficacious in antibiotic prophylaxis. A first- or second-generation cephalosporin such as cephalothin or cefazolin may be substituted for the methicillin and penicillin with slightly reduced coverage. To date, the third-generation cephalosporins have not been found to have adequate ocular penetration and are not appropriate substitutes.

Controversy also surrounds the length of antibiotic treatment. Again, while no clinical trial is available, a four-day course of IV therapy has proven efficacious in the prevention of infections. At the end of this period, all antibiotics are discontinued, and the patient is observed for 24 to 48 hours. If there is still no sign of infection, the patient is discharged from the hospital on no antibiotics.

d. Preoperative Checklist

A checklist of preoperative measures is given in Table 8–1. Orders should be written requiring that the patient be given nothing by mouth and that an IV line be started to provide fluid maintenance and a route for antibiotics.

A protective shield is placed over the eye and a moistened eyepad is used if there are lacerations of the lids that need to be kept moist until repair. Special care must be taken to ensure that no pressure is transmitted to the lacerated globe. For instance, if the patient needs x-rays and the radiology technician is unfamiliar with the care of such patients, the ophthalmologist should accompany the patient to the radiology suite and personally handle the dressings.

Appropriate preoperative laboratory tests should be ordered, and arrangements should be made for any needed radiologic studies. Tetanus prophylaxis should be ordered according to the immunization history of the patient (Table 8–2).

General anesthesia is virtually mandatory to avoid dangerous orbital pressure on the globe from the use of retrobulbar anesthesia, even without an induced retrobulbar hemorrhage. The anesthesiologist should be notified immediately that a case must be scheduled and the operating room staff alerted as well. There is no evidence that a delay of a few hours will adversely affect the final visual outcome, but common sense dictates that the repair should be carried out as soon as feasible. However, the delay of several hours to obtain the necessary laboratory and radiologic tests necessary to adequately evaluate the patient's condition is almost always justified. In addition, if the surgeon needs to have more expert assistance

Table 8–1. PREOPERATIVE CHECKLIST

1. History
2. Physical examination.
3. Cultures.
4. Shield.
5. Nothing by mouth (NPO).
6. Antibiotics.
7. Tetanus toxoid.
8. Preop lab tests.
9. X-rays.
10. Notify anesthesia and operating room staff.

Table 8–2. GUIDE TO TETANUS PROPHYLAXIS IN WOUND MANAGEMENT

History of Tetanus Immunization (Doses)	Clean Minor Wounds		All Other Wounds	
	Tetanus Toxoid	Tetanus Immune Globulin (Human)	Tetanus Toxoid	Tetanus Immune Globulin (Human)
Uncertain	Yes	No	Yes	Yes
0 to 1	Yes	No	Yes	Yes
2	Yes	No	Yes	No*
3 or more	No**	No	No†	No

Source: From U.S. Public Health Service, Advisory Committee on Immunization Practices. *Morbidity and Mortality Weekly Report, Supplement.* Vol. 21, No. 25, June 24, 1972. Atlanta, Center for Disease Control.
*Unless wound is more than 24 hours old.
**Unless more than ten years since last dose.
†Unless more than five years since last dose.

than is available in the middle of the night, it is reasonable to delay the case until morning. Such a delay will often result in a better repair and may even prevent complications that would require future additional surgical procedures.

The anesthesiologist should be told of the exact nature of the injury, as the choice of anesthetic agents will be determined by this information. Depolarizing agents such as succinylcholine must be avoided, as they cause an initial contraction of the rectus muscles, which can result in extrusion of intraocular contents.

Finally, written informed consent must be obtained prior to the use of any narcotic analgesics. Any procedures that are planned or that are possible should be specified on the consent form. If the patient is a minor, the examiner needs to obtain the consent of a parent or guardian. If the patient is inebriated, this should be noted in the medical record, and if another opportunity to obtain a consent arises after the patient becomes sober, this should be done. Occasionally, the ophthalmologist is called upon to operate on an unconscious patient. In this case, the rules that govern such surgery are dictated by the local hospital administration.

8.4 CLOSURE OF CORNEAL AND SCLERAL LACERATIONS

Prior to any surgical procedure, the surgeon must outline the goals of therapy for that operation (Table 8–3). These goals, in order of importance, guide the surgeon during the operation. These will be discussed sequentially below.

The patient is brought to the operating room and placed under general anesthesia. The eyelashes are carefully cut with scissors dipped

Table 8–3. GOALS OF THERAPY IN REPAIR OF CORNEAL AND SCLERAL LACERATIONS

1. Close all lacerations.
2. Restore normal intraocular pressure.
3. Avoid incarceration of tissue in wounds.
4. Restore and protect visual axis.

in petrolatum ointment. The lashes stick to the ointment and are therefore not allowed access to the globe. A microscope is then positioned for use during the operation.

The periorbital area is carefully scrubbed, and the conjunctiva is gently irrigated. Sterile drapes are placed over the patient in the routine manner. Silk sutures may be placed through the lid margins for retraction, but a lid speculum is preferable and is usually adequate. Unless topical antibiotics have been used, it is prudent to culture any prolapsed intraocular contents.

a. Closing All Lacerations

If none of the other goals of the operation can be met, the surgeon should not leave the operating room until he is certain that the ocular coats have been sealed. With current microsurgical techniques, even lacerations in the extreme posterior sclera can be closed.

Prior to closing the lacerations, the sclera is explored in any quadrant in which a perforation could possibly be present. A conjunctival peritomy and scleral exploration is so benign that it should be done extensively so as not to miss any ocular penetration. An otherwise perfectly performed repair can eventuate in disaster if any lacerations are left unsutured. The conjunctiva must be removed at its insertion in the cornea and from the cut edge of any scleral laceration. Failure to carefully clean the sclera is a sure way to miss a small perforation.

Conjunctiva. Every conjunctival laceration potentially overlies, and may conceal, a scleral laceration or rupture. Associated conjunctival hemorrhage and edema may obscure the presence of transparent, gelatinous vitreous, black uveal tissue, or gray, slimelike retina, any of which may have herniated through a scleral laceration. Consequently, almost every conjunctival laceration deserves careful visual and instrumental exploration with the patient under topical anesthesia (general anesthesia in uncooperative patients). Dissection of the conjunctiva and Tenon's fascia (Figure 8–12) off of the sclera will determine whether it has been lacerated, punctured, or ruptured.

Instruments suitably delicate for the dissecting task are fine-toothed forceps and spring-action scissors. *As in any ocular manipulation, care must be exercised to eliminate any pressure on the globe, as this may lead to prolapse*

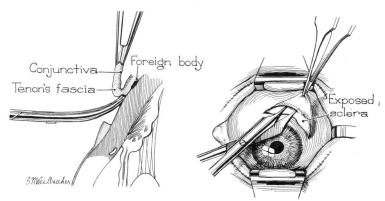

Figure 8–12. Removal of a subconjunctival foreign body requires careful inspection of the globe for possible perforation. Where there is chemosis or hemorrhage, it is easier to get good visualization of the globe by starting the dissection from a nearby incision rather than directly over the foreign body.

of intraocular contents through an unsuspected scleral perforation. If a laceration of the globe is detected at the time of this exploration, it is desirable to proceed immediately with all necessary surgical repairs; thus the operating room should be ready for a more extensive procedure.

The possibility that occult foreign bodies may be buried under a flap of torn and hemorrhagic conjunctiva must always be similarly considered. *As with all foreign bodies removed from the eye and adnexa, the material should be cultured for bacterial and fungal growth rather than taped to the patient's chart.* If exposed intraocular tissue is discovered, it should be manipulated as little as possible and should be prevented from bulging into the scleral wound.

Healing of conjunctival lacerations is remarkably rapid and usually free from infection. Therefore, surgical repair is rarely necessary when such lacerations are less than 1 cm in length. However, prophylactic use of topical antibiotic drops or ointment is advisable for the few days necessary for wound sealing. In the event that surgical reapproximation of lacerated conjunctiva is undertaken, interrupted or continuous 6-0 or 7-0 gut or 8-0 collagen sutures are sufficient. Only two precautions bear mentioning. Since lacerated conjunctival edges are frequently thin, translucent, and rolled or inverted (Figure 8–13), careful recognition and reapproximation of these edges are required to prevent inclusion of Tenon's fascia in the wound or implantation of conjunctival epithelium in the subconjunctival space. The former surgical imperfection leads to a chalky white herniation, and the latter may produce inclusion cyst formation. Knowledge of the normal anatomy of the plica semilunaris and the caruncle (see Figure 8–13) is required to prevent an unsightly surgical repair. Traction on the plica by tight closure of inadequately immobilized

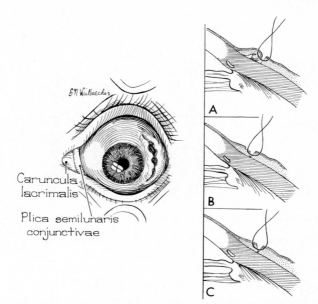

Figure 8–13. Normal conjunctival anatomy and suturing technique for extensive conjunctival lacerations. Small conjunctival lacerations need not be sutured. The caruncle and plica should be preserved whenever possible. (A) Incorrect suture placement with inverted conjunctiva will lead to development of inclusion cysts. (B) Improper suture placement will allow herniation of Tenon's fascia into the wound. (C) Correct suture placement. When extensive destruction or loss of conjunctiva has occurred, bare sclera is distinctly preferable to mucous membrane grafting, particularly when conjunctiva has been lost through injury and the wound is contaminated. This is not the case, however, with severe chemical injuries.

bulbar conjunctiva may produce a disfiguring appearance of the nasal portion of the eye, particularly in terms of redness from the rich blood supply of the plica tissue that is normally in a retracted position near the caruncle.

Sclera. The key steps in the repair of corneoscleral lacerations are outlined in Table 8–4. In general, it is easiest to close the scleral wounds first. Prior to any manipulation, however, the surgeon should create an

Table 8–4. STEPS IN REPAIR OF CORNEOSCLERAL LACERATIONS

1. Make stab incision into anterior chamber.
2. Place traction sutures.
3. Perform conjunctival peritomy.
4. Approximate limbus.
5. Repair scleral lacerations.
6. Remove muscles if necessary.
7. Perform cryotherapy or diathermy if wound extends beyond ora serrata.
8. Repair corneal lacerations.
9. Sweep iris from corneal wound.

incision into the anterior chamber for later access. The anterior chamber is often formed at the beginning of the case, and the tract is created early before the chamber shallows during the manipulation necessary to close the scleral wounds.

It is often advantageous to place sutures through the limbal tissue for traction. This is best done early in the case. A 6-0 silk suture can easily be placed at the two poles 90 degrees from the scleral laceration. In other words, if the laceration on the sclera extends posteriorly from the 3 o'clock position, the sutures are placed at 12 and 6 o'clock. They are then clamped together on a hemostat and the eye rotated to reveal the laceration.

If the laceration involves the limbus, this must be reapproximated first. When this has been accomplished, the globe will suddenly take on a normal contour. If the laceration runs along the limbus, the entire limbal extent is closed before further dissection.

The sclera is then closed beginning anteriorly and proceeding posteriorly. There is a tendency to use excessively coarse suture material for scleral wounds. The tensile strength of 8-0 silk is sufficient for most repairs, although 7-0 silk or 6-0 synthetic sutures are entirely acceptable provided a spatula needle is used. Indeed, many ophthalmic trauma surgeons prefer 9-0 nylon suture to close small scleral lacerations. Occasionally, a few 6-0 silk sutures will bring a gaping wound together so that it can be finished with 8-0 silk. The 6-0 sutures can then either be replaced or left in the sclera for added wound security.

Commonly, especially in the face of a rupture of the sclera, the wound extends circumferentially along the limbus and then radially in the direction of a rectus muscle. Lines of rupture are apparently set up by the tension of the muscular contractions. If the laceration extends to the insertion of a rectus muscle, the muscle should be mobilized with two single-armed 5-0 Vicryl or Dexon sutures and then disinserted. (One must never assume that the rupture ends at the insertion.)

When the end of the scleral laceration is identified and the extent of the wound has been repaired, the length is measured as well as its distance from the limbus. If the surgeon suspects that the laceration may overlie the ora serrata or retina (remember that the ora serrata is roughly at the level of the insertion of the rectus muscles), a single or double row of partially penetrating scleral diathermy should be placed around the sutured wound to obtain a firm retinal adhesion. Alternatively, the wound may be frozen with a cryoprobe. Single freezes to $-60°$ C are sufficient.

If the wound is far posterior, and especially if vitreous has been lost, consideration may be given to buckling the sclera at the time of primary wound repair. The rationale for such an approach is the prevention of vitreous traction and subsequent retinal detachment. Scleral exoplant procedures using silicone rubber sponges are particularly well suited for this type of injury. As in all cases of retinal perforation, placement of the diathermy or cryotherapy probe (after completion of the laceration repair) is precisely accomplished when simultaneous observation with an indirect ophthalmoscope is possible. Hemorrhage or cataract may prevent such precision. The subject of primary vitrectomy in such cases is discussed below.

Scleral lacerations associated with loss of tissue or with wound edges sufficiently damaged to prevent proper apposition can be repaired by means of a hinged scleral flap (Figure 8–14) or a patch graft, using freehand-cut donor material (Figure 8–15). Lacerated tissue should not be excised but should be incorporated into the repair.

Vitreous and uvea are often encountered while repairing the sclera. Ciliary body and choroid should be reposited unless it is grossly contaminated or severely traumatized. In such an event, the excision should be made after encircling the portion to be excised with trans-scleral diathermy, not only to minimize the possibility of subsequent uveal detachment[2] but also to minimize bleeding when the excision is performed. Such eyes have a severely guarded prognosis for salvage, even though partial cyclectomy or choroidectomy is usually successful when employed in nontraumatized eyes for *en bloc* excision of uveal tumors. The eye must

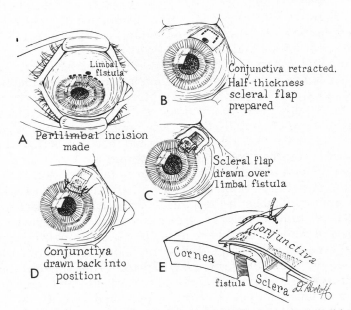

Figure 8–14. Stab wounds at the limbus and scleral defects can be repaired in a manner similar to the technique described for the management of a chronic limbal fistula. The limbus-based hinged scleral flap is drawn over the excised fistula and secured to superficial cornea. (This figure published with the permission of Maumenee AE, Paton D, Morse P, Butner R: Epithelial downgrowth following cataract extraction: a review of 40 histologically proven cases and description of suggested surgical management. Am J Ophthalmol 69:598–603, 1970.)

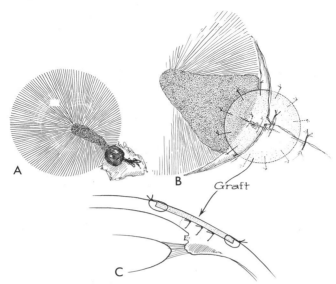

Figure 8–15. (A) Limbal laceration caused by broken glass 12 hours prior to surgery. Preoperative examination showed no evidence of lens damage; prolapsed uveal tissue contained fine bits of glass on its surface. (B) At the time of repair, the prolapsed iris was excised and ciliary body reposited. However, when the sutures used to close the scleral portion of the laceration were tied tightly enough to close the jagged wound, the normal ocular contour dimpled, suggesting that avulsion or loss of some tissue had occurred. Thus, the sutures were removed and replaced with absorbable sutures tight enough only to restore normal contour. Air was injected into the anterior chamber. A 6-mm trephine mark was made to center the laceration and straddle the limbus. All remnants of Tenon's fascia were removed from this trephined bed. Corneal-episcleral lamellar dissection was carried out from the periphery toward the center of the marked surface for a distance sufficient to establish a sharp-margined recipient bed for placement of a glycerin-preserved lamellar donor graft of corneal tissue. Diathermy was placed around the scleral laceration. (C) The graft was secured with multiple interrupted sutures. The conjunctiva was then closed over the peripheral portion of the graft. The graft opacified; fibrous tissue bridged and healed the scleral laceration. It is a rare injury that requires donor tissue for primary repair.

be evaluated carefully before the seventh to tenth postoperative days to decide if the globe is salvageable or if it should be enucleated to minimize the chance of sympathetic ophthalmia. Vitreous should be touched with a cellulose sponge and amputated. This methodical technique will sometimes ultimately result in the vitreous body falling away from the wound. Automated vitrectomy instruments should not be inserted into the wound, as the intraocular structures cannot be visualized and the possibility of damaging the lens or retina is great. The use of vitrectomy instrumentation is discussed later in this chapter.

The prolapse of retina through a scleral laceration is a very poor prognostic sign, and such eyes are almost invariably lost. If retinal prolapse is suspected, a small biopsy may be sent for subsequent documentation.

If the biopsy reveals retinal tissue, the patient must often be scheduled for enucleation, as the prospect of achieving useful visual acuity is low.

Cornea. Prior to beginning repair of the corneal laceration, great care must be taken to ensure that the laceration does not involve the sclera. If the laceration approaches the limbus, a conjunctival peritomy must be made in that area and the sclera carefully inspected. *Never assume that a laceration that seems to stop at the limbus has not extended into the sclera.*

The major advantage of proceeding to repair of a corneal laceration without delay is the avoidance of tissue edema, which makes the repair progressively more difficult as the hours pass. Fine suture material such as 9-0 or 10-0 nylon will tend to loosen in the postoperative period unless the suture loop extends well beyond the area of edema on both sides of the wound. Generally, interrupted sutures taking 1- to 2-mm bites from each lip of the wound can repair a clear corneal laceration if minimal edema is present.

Marked edema necessitates tissue bites of up to 2.5 mm on each side. In the latter circumstance, needles of greater radius of curvature must be selected, for the surgeon should always attempt to place the suture by completing the arc of the needle's curvature rather than by dragging the needle through the tissue to make a bite wider than the small arc of the needle's curvature permits. Figure 8–16 indicates recommended variations in tissue depth and width for suture bites under different circumstances of corneal injury. The depth of most sutures should be two thirds to three quarters of corneal thickness. However, on completion of a laceration repair and despite normal contour of the cornea, occasional wound leakage occurs that can be cured by a few superficial sutures. These sutures may or may not be extruded spontaneously. Such "final" interrupted sutures will facilitate the closure and will make replacement of other well-located sutures unnecessary.

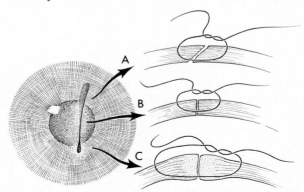

Figure 8–16. Repair of corneal laceration. The diagram illustrates suggested placement of nylon suture material. (A) For shelved laceration. (B) For vertical laceration. (C) For laceration with edematous margins.

If possible, 10-0 nylon sutures should be used to close the cornea. These leave only a minimal scar and are usually strong enough to hold the wound edges in place. Occasionally, if the cornea is very edematous or if the wound is very long, 9-0 nylon sutures may be used. In some cases, several 9-0 sutures are used to reapproximate the wound, and then the spaces between them are closed with 10-0 nylon. In general, it is prudent to place the first suture in the center of the laceration and then to sequentially divide each half of the remaining unsutured laceration until the wound is tight.

The surgeon should minimize trauma to corneal tissue by precise suturing that does not require more than occasional replacement of sutures during the operative procedure. There are three basic types of corneal lacerations: linear, jagged, and stellate (puncture wounds). Although a continuous nylon suture can be used to close a clean, straight corneal laceration, particularly if the wound runs through the visual axis, interrupted sutures are advisable in most circumstances, as they can be removed one at a time and if one loosens or breaks the others will remain intact. The suture ends should be cut short with a razor knife, but the knots should not be buried, as this makes removal more difficult. Corneal epithelium quickly covers the knots, and discomfort is rarely a problem after a few days.

For jagged lacerations, the closure is comparable to that advocated for linear lacerations, except that continuous sutures can never be employed in such cases, and the task of obtaining ideal reapproximation of tissues is more difficult. Stellate lacerations usually occur from a puncture wound and may be associated with foreign bodies retained in areas such as the anterior chamber, the lens, or the vitreous cavity. A puncture wound may be extremely small, yet sufficient to introduce surface epithelium, causing late occurrence of an epithelial cyst of the iris; there is no known prophylaxis for such unusual late complications (Figure 8–17). One such case involving a puncture wound occurred at the time of prenatal amniocentesis.[3]

Closure of a stellate laceration can be difficult. The absence of marked tissue edema may allow the use of interrupted and/or purse-string suture techniques (Figure 8–18). When a small amount of corneal tissue has been destroyed or lost, a cyanoacrylate monomer can be used to seal the lesion in many cases.[4] The glue is drawn into a syringe through a 25-gauge needle, and then a small drop is expelled so that it sits on the tip of the needle. The assistant then dries the area of the perforation and the drop of glue is quickly placed on the site. Care must be taken to place the glue on a completely dry surface or it will not seal the wound. The surface hardens in 30 seconds, and the edges are inspected to detect any lifting off of the glue from the corneal surface (Figure 8–19). A bandage contact lens is then placed over the cornea for comfort and to protect the glue

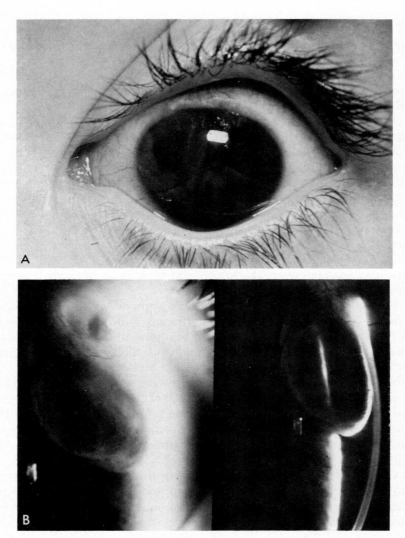

Figure 8–17. (A) Perforating injuries can lead to the late occurrence of epithelial cysts of the iris, as shown in this eye of a 10-year-old boy who had sustained a stab injury from a dart five years earlier. (B) A similar, but single-lobed, epithelial cyst of the iris occurred in the eye of a 14-year-old boy two years following a laceration of the limbus. Two views of the cyst are shown.

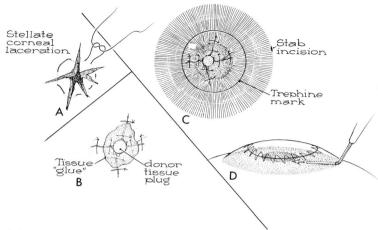

Figure 8–18. (A) A stellate laceration of the cornea can be closed by a single purse-string suture when there is no loss of tissue, or (B) with the additional use of cyanoacrylate monomer and even a plug of donor corneal tissue. However, when such lesions are central, and particularly if the lens has been injured, it is better to follow preliminary closure of the wound by (C) penetrating keratoplasty. A stab incision is made at the limbus and the anterior chamber filled (D) with balanced salt solution or air if necessary. A trephine mark is made on the cornea and the button excised. After lens removal, and vitrectomy if necessary (see Figure 8–20), a graft is secured in the recipient trephined bed. The anterior chamber is refilled with balanced salt solution.

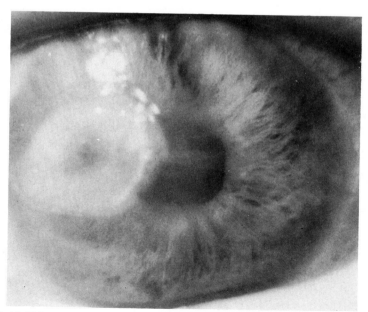

Figure 8–19. This patient's corneal injury has been repaired by the use of a patch graft and cyanoacrylate monomer. Ultimately, penetrating keratoplasty will be required if the eye is to regain good visual acuity.

from being wiped off during eyelid movements. Occasionally, it is impossible to dry the area. The anterior chamber may be filled with air or hyaluronic acid (Healon or Amvisc), which will sometimes provide a dry bed on which to work.[5]

Supplementary use of a patch graft or freehand-cut donor corneal tissue is helpful in closing large or irregular defects from tissue loss.[6] Alternatively, the use of conjunctival flaps is a tried and true method for sealing irregular corneal lacerations. A full-thickness pedicle of conjunctiva with Tenon's fascia can be drawn over the laceration and secured at this site. Such a pedicle will retract within days or weeks, by which time tissue fibrosis may have been sufficient to seal the wound.

The use of a corneal graft in the primary repair of an ocular injury is rarely necessary. Large stellate lacerations, however, should be repaired primarily by partial penetrating keratoplasty (Figure 8–20; see also Figure 8–18). The trephine employed should be large enough to cover all abnormal tissue; if possible, the margin of the graft should not cross the visual axis. Initially, the globe should be sutured sufficiently to establish the best possible approximation of normal corneal contours before the trephine is used to mark the corneal tissue. A suction trephine (Hessberg-Barron) is now available that facilitates trephination in these soft eyes.

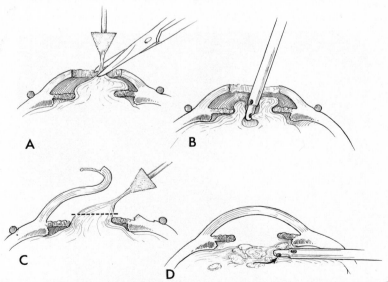

Figure 8–20. This figure summarizes four basic techniques for performing vitrectomy. Choice of technique depends on the individual requirements of the injured eye and the availability of instrumentation. (A) The Kasner technique of performing a vitrectomy with cellulose sponge through a trephined corneal defect prior to keratoplasty. (B) Vitrectomy performed with a vitreous suction-cutter through a corneal laceration. (C) Kasner technique for vitrectomy performed through a large limbal incision after previous repair of a corneal laceration. (D) Lensectomy and vitrectomy performed with a vitreous suction-cutter instrument introduced through the pars plana.

Even though the anterior chamber has been entered, shelving lacerations may be self-sealing, and the anterior chamber may be fully reformed by the time of initial examination. If the wound is well approximated and appears to be stable, the only therapy required may be the use of a patch and shield. However, if there is any question about the stability of the wound, a suture should be placed through it. In any case, any time the inside of the eye has been penetrated, IV antibiotics are indicated. There are many reports of self-sealing corneal lacerations proceeding to purulent endophthalmitis.

When a corneal wound appears to be self-sealing, a Seidel test is helpful in confirming the presence or absence of leakage. Highly concentrated (2%) sodium fluorescein is placed on the wound and the area carefully observed. If a leak exists, the aqueous will dilute the concentrated fluorescein, resulting in a stream of green (dilute) fluorescein within a field of orange (concentrated) solution. The use of moistened fluorescein strips is a poor alternative, as the dye is less concentrated and there is a higher chance of false negative result.

Corneal lacerations that are only partially penetrating rarely need to be sutured. If the laceration is not self-sealing, if it extends through more than 50 per cent of the corneal stroma, or if it is more than 3 to 4 mm long, primary closure with appositional sutures should be considered. Small corneal lacerations may be effectively splinted, without suturing, by means of a soft contact lens.

In repair of any corneal laceration, the number of sutures placed directly in the visual axis should be limited, although this concern is secondary in importance to good tissue apposition (Figure 8–21). The knots create scars that are more visually important than the rest of the wound. Therefore, if the laceration is near the visual axis, all knots should be rotated away from the center of the pupil, and if it goes through the axis, the knots should be alternated so that every second knot is on the same side of the wound.

b. Restoring Normal Intraocular Pressure

Most eyes with perforating injuries are mushy soft, and this status will persist until the laceration has been closed and the normal ocular volume reconstituted. It is important to re-form the anterior chamber during the surgical repair to restore normal ocular contours. For this purpose, air is more effective than saline. A large bubble of air also delineates the presence and location of vitreous in the anterior chamber: the vitreous will deform the air bubble. The dangers of air-block glaucoma and the adhesions that can occur in the chamber angle when air gets behind the iris are obvious. Air is useful during operative repair, but most of it should be replaced by a balanced salt solution before the surgery is completed.

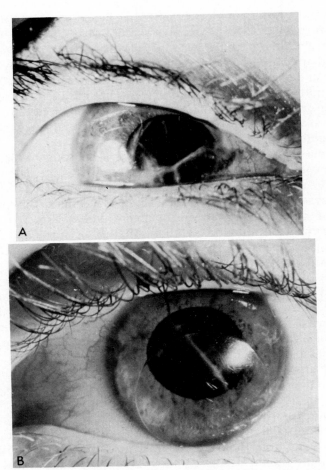

Figure 8–21. Repaired and healed corneal lacerations often permit good postoperative vision. (A) 20/40 with spectacle correction. (B) 20/30 in another case with contact lens. Thus, avoid keratoplasty as part of primary procedure whenever possible.

When the eye is soft, it is sometimes difficult to make a stab incision at the limbus or pars plana. A large-toothed forceps used to grasp the eye next to the intended site of entry is helpful, and the use of a very sharp disposable knife is essential. Ideally, the incision is made at the beginning of the operation, before the anterior chamber has become flattened by manipulation of the globe. The incision should be beveled so that it is self-sealing or at most requires only one suture to be closed.

In restoring the normal intraocular pressure it must be kept in mind that the pressure in the anterior chamber may not instantly equilibrate with the pressure in the vitreous chamber. The anterior chamber is first filled with balanced salt solution, and the corneal suture line is checked to be sure that it is water tight. If hyaluronic acid has previously been used to reform the chamber, the wound must be inspected very carefully, for this viscous solution may give the surgeon a false sense of security that the wound is tight. The scleral wound is then inspected for water tightness. If the sclera is slightly collapsed, the vitreous may be re-formed through an injection of balanced salt solution or air given through the para plana 3.5 mm from the limbus. This maneuver is fraught with danger, however, since the ciliary body may be detached, and the injection may be unwittingly given in the suprachoroidal space, resulting in a total detachment of the choroid and retina.

c. Avoiding Tissue Incarceration in the Wound

When iris is incarcerated in the depths of a corneal laceration, the tissue should be swept into its normal position. This is performed most conveniently with a fine iris spatula or "sweep" manipulated through the stab incision made at the beginning of the operation. Ideally, the incision has been made about 60 degrees away from the edge of the laceration and points toward the laceration. In this way, only minimal distortion of the incision will be necessary during the sweeping maneuver. Often, a single sweep is done and then one or more corneal sutures can be placed. A second sweep is then done and the laceration is finally closed with additional sutures. If the anterior chamber is flat, it should be re-formed with air, balanced salt solution, or hyaluronic acid prior to the sweeping, as the instrument might otherwise damage the corneal endothelium or the lens. Occasionally, the initial sutures cannot be placed without sweeping and in addition the anterior chamber cannot be deepened without some sutures in the wound. In this case, the assistant can place a spatula along the length of the wound, forcing the iris into the eye, and the surgeon can then place a suture through the lips of the wound over the instrument. Once one or two such sutures are closing the wound, the chamber can usually be formed (Figures 8–22 through 8–27).

Avoidance of incarceration of tissues into a scleral wound is usually less of a problem and is also probably less important. In general, the technique just described in which the assistant incorporates the uvea under the wound while the surgeon places a suture is very successful. In addition, the surgeon may wish to place the suture through one lip of the wound, then pull the needle through and reposition it in the needle holder before approaching the other lip of the wound. Often, the needle can be "walked down" the wall of the second edge of the sclera, with the curve of the needle pushing the uvea down and away from the tip. In this way, the tip never passes through uvea that is not, therefore, incarcerated into the wound.

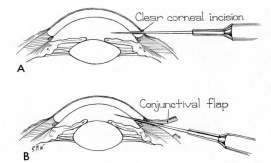

Figure 8–22. Techniques of performing surgical stab incisions at the limbus. (A) Ziegler knife enters the anterior chamber through clear cornea at the limbus. (B) With a shallow anterior chamber, the Ziegler knife puncture is made under a conjunctival flap with the blade parallel to the surface of the iris. In both cases, the tip of the blade must be directed away from the lens and iris, but not so far forward that the corneal endothelium is touched.

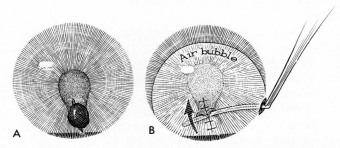

Figure 8–23. Corneal laceration with iris prolapse, small hyphema, and undamaged lens. This recently lacerated eye is managed by an initial stab incision at the limbus (Ziegler knife), preliminary sweeping of the iris toward the pupil to reduce the prolapse, injection of air into the anterior chamber, repair of laceration with interrupted 10–0 nylon sutures, further reduction of any recurrent iris adhesion, and (B) final evacuation of air and replacement by balanced salt solution.

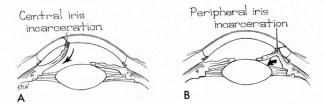

Figure 8–24. The pharmacologic means used to reduce a recent and minimal iris adhesion to a corneal wound depend on the location of the wound. (A) Topically applied atropine is sometimes useful in central incarcerations because of its action in dilating the pupil (arrow). (B) Pilocarpine or other miotics occasionally constrict the pupil enough to pull the iris free (arrow), but surgery is required if these means fail. At surgery, the iris should be swept from the periphery toward the central portion of the anterior chamber. There should be minimal manipulation of iris tissue and care taken not to touch the lens or corneal endothelium.

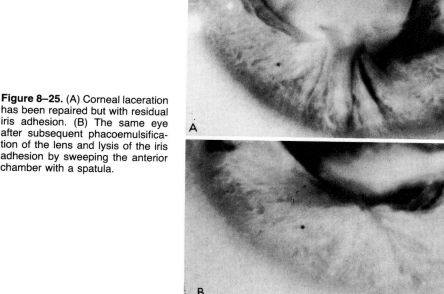

Figure 8–25. (A) Corneal laceration has been repaired but with residual iris adhesion. (B) The same eye after subsequent phacoemulsification of the lens and lysis of the iris adhesion by sweeping the anterior chamber with a spatula.

As stated previously, if the scleral laceration extends beyond the ora serrata (roughly at the level of the insertion of the rectus muscles), transscleral diathermy or cryotherapy over the repaired laceration should be employed.

8.5 LENS DAMAGE ASSOCIATED WITH PERFORATING INJURIES

If definite laceration of the lens accompanies an ocular perforation, lens surgery often can be accomplished at the time of the primary repair. However, unless the lens is cataractous or is observed in the preoperative period to be becoming progressively more opaque, it is difficult to predict the degree of visual disability it may cause. Removal of the lens, particularly in a child, in whom aphakic correction is difficult, is not a benign treatment. Although the surgery is often not technically difficult, the postoperative course is many times frustrating for the patient and doctor. Physicians commonly underestimate the difficulties of aphakic contact lenses, especially in the presence of corneal scars. Caution, therefore, should be exercised before opting for removal of the lens.

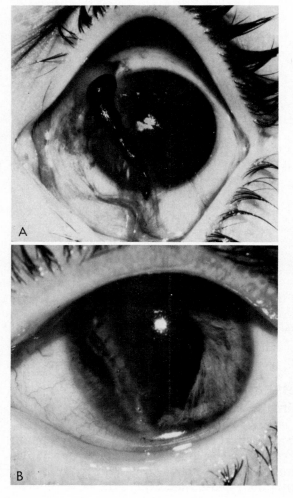

Figure 8–26. (A) Corneoscleral laceration without damage to the lens. (B) The same eye after excision of iris prolapse and repair of the laceration.

Figure 8–27. (A) Corneoscleral laceration has been repaired with wide excision of prolapsed iris and lavage of a cataract at the time of primary repair. Vitreous loss necessitated an anterior vitrectomy. Postoperatively, the intraocular pressure was normal, but the acuity was limited to finger counting owing to the corneal scarring. (B) The same eye after secondary repair, demonstrating how severely traumatized eyes can be salvaged. A partial penetrating keratoplasty was performed, lens remnants and more vitreous were removed, and the large coloboma of the iris was also repaired with two interrupted 10–0 nylon sutures. Postoperatively, the aphakic vision was 20/30, but the patient developed a rhegmatogenous retinal detachment necessitating repair. The graft remains clear, the retina is now flat, and there is an encircling element producing a moderately high buckle.

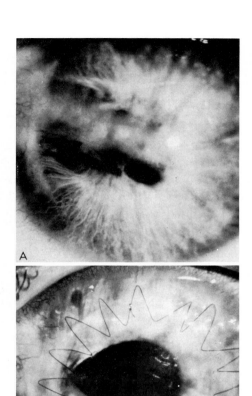

Evaluation of the patient for primary lens removal is often difficult. Particularly in children, a marked fibrinoid reaction in the anterior chamber appearing as a dense cloud on the lens surface can obscure a view of the lens capsule and may simulate flocculent lens material. Free and partially clotted blood also can obscure a sufficient view of the lens necessary to make a judgment as to whether it is cataractous. In addition, vitreous hemorrhage frequently gives a reflection on the posterior lens capsule that can appear to be a significant capsular opacity.

When there is a large laceration of the cornea and when the surgeon can be certain that the vitreous is undisturbed, flocculent lens material can be aspirated through the corneal wound itself (Figures 8–28 and 8–29). However, in most cases complete removal of lens substance will necessitate a surgical incision at the limbus or in the pars plana once the corneal laceration has been repaired (Figures 8–30 and 8–31). If the surgeon is familiar with extracapsular cataract removal, it is usually most convenient to repair the corneal laceration first and then make a standard cataract wound and aspirate the lens. If the patient is too old to aspirate the nucleus, phacoemulsification may be useful.

8.6 LACERATIONS INVOLVING THE VITREOUS

The most dangerous lacerations are those that involve the lens, ciliary body, and vitreous.[7–9] Just a few years ago it was classic teaching to recommend enucleation of eyes with poor light projection following repair of perforating injuries that had caused damage to the lens and vitreous.

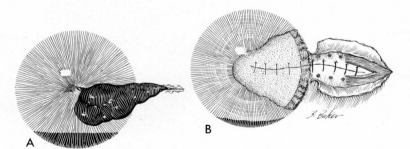

Figure 8–28. (A) Corneoscleral laceration with iris prolapse and damage to the lens. The steps of surgical repair are as follows: (1) bulbar conjunctival dissection to determine extent of scleral laceration, (2) excision of iris prolapse in this patient with lens injury, (3) preliminary removal of extruding lens material through lacerations, (4) first laceration suture placed at limbus, (5) partial closure of corneal laceration and closure of scleral laceration, (6) aspiration and irrigation of lens material through corneal wound (if readily accomplished), (7) completion of corneal wound closure with interrupted 10–0 nylon sutures, (8) re-formation of anterior chamber with balanced salt solution, (9) microsurgical inspection to determine adequacy of lens substance removal, most probably followed by separate stab incisions at the limbus for irrigation and aspiration of additional lens material, (10) partial penetrating diathermy *surrounding* scleral portion of laceration, and (11) closure of conjunctival defect. The completed repair is shown in (B).

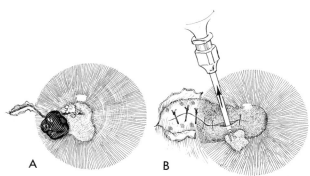

Figure 8–29. (A) Extensive corneoscleral laceration with iris and ciliary body prolapse and hyphema. The steps of surgical repair are as follows: (1) exploration of the extent of scleral laceration and hemostasis, (2) excision of prolapsed iris and reposition of ciliary body, (3) inspection for damage to lens, (4) repair of corneoscleral laceration starting at limbus, (5) reformation of anterior chamber with balanced salt solution injected through separate stab incision, (6) diathermy to injured ciliary body surrounding scleral laceration, (7) repair of conjunctival defect, and (8) no further surgery if lens is intact. (B) Aspiration of flocculent lens fragments. This is performed uncommonly, because fibrinous aqueous may sometimes mimic lens fragments, and the obscured lens may in actuality be intact. If one is completely certain that the lens is grossly lacerated, one can aspirate it at the time of surgery as shown here or by way of a separate pars plana incision and the vitrophage, as illustrated in Figure 8–31.

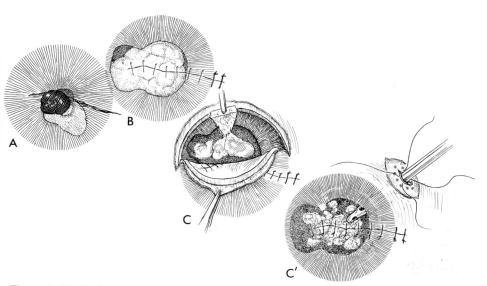

Figure 8–30. (A) Corneoscleral laceration with iris, lens, and vitreous prolapse. The steps of surgical repair are as follows: (1) exploration of the extent of scleral laceration, (2) excision of iris, lens, and vitreous prolapse sufficient to permit partial formation of anterior chamber using air, (3) closure of corneoscleral laceration (B) with interrupted sutures, using air and then balanced salt solution for normalizing ocular contour, (4) wide cataract section under conjunctival flap (C) to lay back repaired cornea, followed by removal of lens material and vitrectomy, and (5) closure of limbal incision and retesting of both wounds to be sure they are "watertight." Alternatively (C'), the trained surgeon may elect to aspirate lens material and vitreous through the laceration or through a pars plana incision after closure of the corneal laceration. Specialized instrumentation is required.

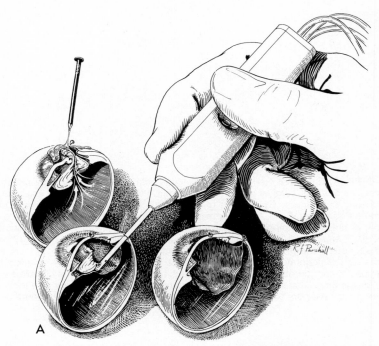

A

Figure 8–31. Techniques employing the vitrophage. (A) Perforation of the eye can result in prolapse of iris, lens, and vitreous. Reconstruction of the anterior segment of the eye can be accomplished with the vitrophage,* even in the immediate post-traumatic period. After closure of the wound of entry, the vitrophage is inserted through a single 3- to 4-mm incision in the pars plana. Aspiration of tissue into the tip of the instrument is achieved when the surgeon closes the aperture on the body of the instrument with his thumb or forefinger. Prolapsed or adherent iris, lens, and vitreous can be bitten out and aspirated in a relatively atraumatic fashion, creating optically clear anterior and posterior chambers. The anterior portion of the vitreous chamber is also rendered clear. It is rarely necessary to include the posterior vitreous gel in this type of vitrectomy.

Illustration continued on opposite page

Now, as ophthalmic trauma surgeons develop more experience with techniques of lens and vitreous removal, many such eyes can be salvaged and restored to useful vision.

There is no agreement among ophthalmic trauma surgeons as to whether it is better to do a vitrectomy as part of the primary repair or to wait several days. The advantages of primary vitrectomy are that there is only one anesthesia and that early removal of the vitreous/lens/blood admixture may prevent a subsequent tractional retinal detachment. In

---

*Peyman GA, Diamond J: The vitrophage in ocular reconstruction following trauma. Can J Ophthalmol *10*:419–422, 1975.

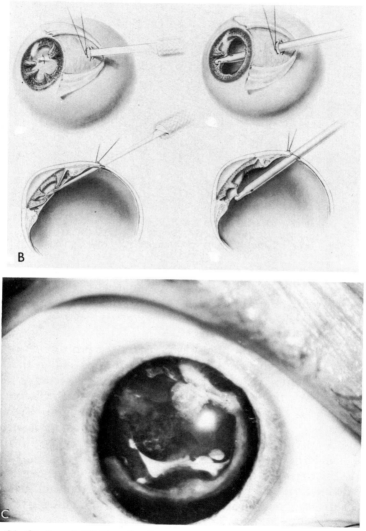

Figure 8–31. *Continued.* (B) The vitrophage can also be used effectively when a traumatic cataract has evolved into a dense secondary pupillary membrane. The two drawings at left show a Beaver 52S disposable blade entering through the pars plana and the secondary membrane. The two drawings at right show a vitrophage taking small bites in membrane and posterior synechias. (C) A secondary membrane 11 years after cataract surgery.

Illustration continued on following page

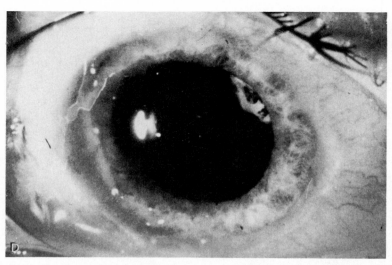

Figure 8–31. *Continued.* (D) View of eye shown in (C) following the operation described in (B). (B), (C), and (D) are from Peyman GA, Swartz M: Management of dense secondary membranes with the vitrophage. Albrecht von Graefe's Arch Klin Ophthalmol *195*:155–159, 1975.

addition, if a retinal detachment has occurred during the initial injury, it can be repaired early, resulting in a theoretically better prognosis for macular vision.[10]

The advantages of vitrectomy as a secondary procedure are equally compelling. Experimental and clinical experience has shown that detachment of the posterior vitreous face occurs seven to ten days following traumatic vitreous hemorrhage.[11] Posterior vitreous detachment clearly makes the surgery technically less difficult. In addition, hypotony is frequently present in the early period after an injury, and this often leads to detachment of the ciliary body. Placement of the vitrectomy instruments into the eye through such a detachment can result in total uveal and retinal detachment. After several days, the ciliary detachments usually resolve, making vitrectomy safer. Finally, a delay of several days allows the cornea to deturgess, resulting in better visualization during the difficult and dangerous vitrectomy procedure.

8.7 SYMPATHETIC OPHTHALMIA

Any perforating injury of the eye (especially with prolapse of the iris or ciliary body) has a slight but significant chance of inducing sympathetic ophthalmia (Figure 8–32). Even subconjunctival rupture caused by a blunt injury of the globe can lead to sympathetic ophthalmia[12] with a severe, bilateral, granulomatous uveitis originating from unilateral injury. With

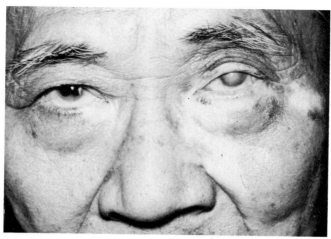

Figure 8–32. Sympathetic ophthalmia. The patient's right eye sustained a perforating injury with damage to the ciliary body. Three months later, sympathetic ophthalmia occurred in the left eye, progressing to a mere light perception despite steroid therapy. Poliosis and vitiligo have accompanied the sympathetic ophthalmia. The injured eye has 20/60 vision.

the greater degree of salvage afforded by modern vitreous surgery, the incidence of this dreaded disorder has not decreased.

Sympathetic ophthalmia is possibly due to injury-induced autosensitivity to uveal tissue, a theory recently revitalized by animal experimentation.[13] In trauma cases in which iris or ciliary body prolapses have not been treated and in which the injured eye has not been enucleated within a week or so after the injury, the incidence of sympathetic ophthalmia may be as high as 3 to 5 per cent.[14] Sympathetic ophthalmia remains a threat to be considered with every injured eye that has been perforated (Figure 8–33).

Sympathetic ophthalmia may occur within one and one half weeks to many years after the initial perforating injury. Eighty per cent of cases occur within three months of injury. It is important to decide within the first five to ten days of the initial injury whether the patient's repaired eye has a fair chance of providing useful vision, for if it does not, enucleation is advisable to prevent sympathetic ophthalmia. Once the second (sympathizing) eye is involved, it is uncertain whether enucleation of the injured (exciting) eye is beneficial.[15] It has long been held that sympathetic ophthalmia is so severe that the eye originally injured may eventually be the patient's better eye, but since the advent of corticosteroids, this may be less often true.

Sympathetic ophthalmia may occur after incomplete enucleation of a severely traumatized globe, just as it may follow evisceration.[16] Thus if a ruptured, lacerated, or otherwise destroyed eye is removed, the surgeon should be certain to excise all uveal tissue.

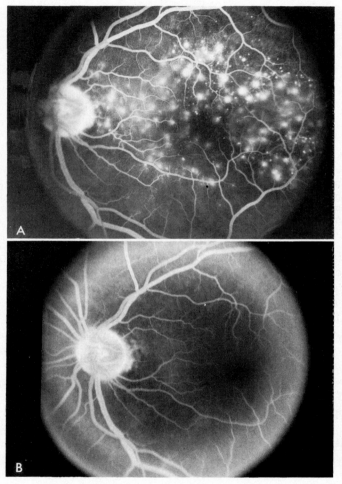

Figure 8–33. (A) Venous phase of fluorescein angiogram in sympathizing eye of patient with histologically confirmed sympathetic ophthalmia. Multiple leaking points in the pigment epithelium are seen and resemble those of Harada's disease. (B) Sympathetic ophthalmia has responded favorably to local and systemic corticosteroids.

References

1. Goldberg MF, Tessler HH: Occult intraocular perforations from brow and lid lacerations. Arch Ophthalmol 86:145–149, 1971.
2. Paton D, Craig J: Management of iridodialysis. Ophthalmic Surg 4(1):38–39, 1973.
3. Cross HE, Maumenee AE: Ocular trauma during amniocentesis. Arch ophthalmol 90:303–304, 1973.
4. Dohlman C: Personal communication, June 1973.
5. Kenyon K: Decision-making in the therapy of external eye disease: Non-infected corneal ulcers. Ophthalmology 89:44–51, 1982.
6. Hyndiuk RA, Hall DS, Kinyoun JL: Free tissue patch and cyanoacrylate in corneal perforations. Ophthalmic Surg 5:50–55, 1974.
7. Coles WH, Haik GM: Vitrectomy in intraocular trauma. Arch Ophthalmol 87:621–628, 1972.
8. Barr CC: Prognostic factors in corneoscleral lacerations. Arch Ophthalmol 101:919–924, 1983.
9. DeJuan E, Sternberg P, Michaels RG; Penetrating ocular injuries: Types of injuries and visual results. Ophthalmology 90:1318–1322, 1983.
10. Coleman DJ: Early vitrectomy in the management of the severely traumatized eye. Am J Ophthalmol 93:543–551, 1982.
11. Ryan SJ, Allen AW: Pars plana vitrectomy in ocular trauma. Am J Ophthalmol 88:483–491, 1979.
12. Baghdassarian SA, Crawford JB, Fine LM: Sympathetic ophthalmia following occult indirect scleral rupture. Surv Ophthalmol 14:327–329, 1970.
13. Wong VG, Anderson R, O'Brien PJ: Sympathetic ophthalmia and lymphocyte transformation. Am J Ophthalmol 72:960–966, 1971.
14. Hogan MJ, Zimmerman LE (eds): Ophthalmic Pathology: An Atlas and Textbook. (Second Edition). Philadelphia, W B Saunders Co, 1962.
15. Lubin JR, Albert DM, Weinstein M: Sixty-five years of sympathetic ophthalmia. A clinicopathologic review of 105 cases (1913–1978). Ophthalmology 87:109–121, 1980.
16. Green WR, Maumenee AE, Saunders T, Smith MS: Sympathetic uveitis following evisceration. Trans Am Acad Ophthalmol Otolaryngol 76:625–644, 1972.

9

Ocular Infections and Antibiotic Therapy

9.1 CULTURE TECHNIQUES

The media and equipment necessary for proper ocular cultures are shown in Figure 9–1. In identifying pathogens, the ophthalmologist must realize the importance of obtaining optimal smears and cultures and transporting them to the laboratory; in turn, the laboratory personnel must be aware of the special aspects of culturing ophthalmic tissue.

There are at least two instances in which it is appropriate to obtain cultures: in the face of an infection, and after a penetrating injury prior to initiating prophylactic therapy. When an infection is present, the principle of "going where the money is" should be observed. In a corneal ulcer, the base and leading edge are cultured; in endophthalmitis, the vitreous and anterior chamber are cultured; in an orbital abscess, the abscess is cultured. After a penetrating injury, an attempt must be made to anticipate the organisms that may cause an ocular infection several days after the injury. The wound may be cultured, as well as the lids, conjunctiva, and the weapon causing the injury if it is available.

Many forms of agar plates and transport media are available. In addition, thioglycollate broth is used to isolate anaerobic and microaerophilic organisms. Sabouraud's agar is very helpful for isolating fungi,

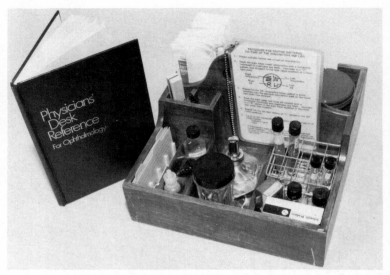

Figure 9–1. The equipment needed for bacteriologic investigation of presumed or known infections of the eye can be contained in a single portable tray. In addition, the ophthalmologist should have a source book available containing information about ophthalmic drugs and their dosages, toxicities, and incompatibilities.

although fungi often grow on standard media as well. Transport media that require only small quantities of ocular fluids have proven of great value in the management of endophthalmitis.

a. Corneal Ulcers

A Gram's stain; a stain for morphology such as Wright's, Giemsa, or Diff Quik*; and a culture of the ulcer are all necessary in the workup of corneal ulcers. A culture of the lids and conjunctiva, while occasionally helpful in sorting out possible contaminants, is rarely helpful in the management of the ulcer. The base and the leading edge are scraped with a Kimura or other platinum spatula that has been flamed. The first material obtained is used to inoculate blood and chocolate agar plates. The spatula is again flamed, and the next material is smeared on two microscope slides, which are then stained with Gram's stain and the morphology stain. Because only a small amount of material is usually obtained, great care must be taken in the fixing of the slide so as not to lose any valuable tissue.

b. Endophthalmitis

When culturing an eye with suspected endophthalmitis, material ordinarily will be obtained from both the vitreous and anterior chambers. While

*Harleco, Gibbstown, New Jersey.

the reason is unknown, samples obtained from the vitreous are more likely to be positive than those obtained from the anterior chamber.[1] For this reason, an anterior chamber tap alone is insufficient in the workup of endophthalmitis.

An assistant receives the sample from the surgeon in a syringe and should attempt to remove all air from the syringe. The contents of the syringe are then inoculated into an anaerobic transport medium (Anaport*). The small amount of fluid that is invariably left in the barrel of the needle is then smeared on two microscope slides. Obviously, it is very important to label the transport vials and the slides so that the aqueous and vitreous samples are not confused. The vitreous samples must dry onto the microscope slides for longer than is routinely allowed in other clinical situations. The process can usually be accelerated by placing the slides into an incubator at 37° C for 15 to 30 minutes.

9.2 TREATMENT OF OCULAR INFECTIONS

The treatment of ocular infections is based on the clinical setting, the results of smears, and the results of cultures. Since the culture results are not available for several hours to several days, the initial therapy must be based on the clinical situation and the smears alone. As both of these are notoriously unreliable, the initial therapy is usually empirical.

a. Post-traumatic Corneal Ulcers

The diagnosis of corneal ulcer is easily made when a portion of the cornea lacks its epithelium (causing fluorescein staining) and is discolored (usually gray, white, or yellow) by the local growth of microorganisms and infiltration of inflammatory cells.[2] A hypopyon (a layer of white blood cells in the anterior chamber) is often present. Bacterial corneal ulceration is the most feared complication of a simple corneal abrasion; therefore, *every patient with an abrasion should be followed until the epithelium is intact.*

Central corneal ulcers are a potential threat to the viability of the eye, and patients with such ulcers should be hospitalized to ensure that antibiotics are given as ordered and the patient is readily available for frequent examinations. Cycloplegics are given to provide patient comfort and to prevent posterior synechia in the miotic position. Elevated intraocular pressure should be medically treated as indicated.

Antibiotic drops are begun using a combination that will provide a broad spectrum of coverage. Cefazolin drops (100 mg/ml) may be alternated with gentamicin drops (3 to 14 mg/ml). Each drug should be given every 30 to 60 minutes so that the patient receives one medication

*Scott Laboratories, Fiskeville, Rhode Island.

Table 9–1. PREPARATION OF ANTIBIOTIC IN TEAR SUBSTITUTES

Antibiotic	Amount in Commercially Prepared Vial	Number of Vials Needed	Diluent Volume Added per Vial	Tear Substitute Volume Removed From 15-ml Drop Applicator	Antibiotic Solution Volume Added to Drop Applicator of Tear Substitute	Final Concentration of Antibiotic
Bacitracin	50,000 units	3	3 ml	9 ml	9 ml (three vials)	10,000 units/ml
Carbenicillin	1000 mg	1	8 ml	None	0.50 ml	4 mg/ml
Neomycin	500 mg	1	4 ml	1 ml	1 ml	8.3 mg/ml
Penicillin G	5 megaunits	1	3 ml	1 ml	1 ml	111,000 units/ml
Vancomycin	500 mg	2	2 ml	3 ml	3 ml (one and one half vials)	50 mg/ml

Source: Prepared from material by Jones DB: Early diagnosis and therapy of bacterial corneal ulcers. Int Ophthalmol Clin 13(4):1–29, 1973.

or the other every 15 to 30 minutes. Other antibiotic combinations include gentamicin and Neosporin, gentamicin and bacitracin, and tobramycin and cephazolin. Some of these solutions are not commercially available as eyedrops and must be produced by the hospital pharmacy (Table 9–1).

There is no advantage of subconjunctival injection over frequent administration of drops.[3] In addition, systemic antibiotics appear to have no place in the management of bacterial corneal ulcers.

b. Endophthalmitis

No infection is more feared by the ophthalmologist than bacterial endophthalmitis (Figure 9–2). Endophthalmitis may not be suspected after trauma, because many of its characteristic clinical signs (lid edema, corneal haze, aqueous or vitreous inflammation, conjunctival hyperemia, and edema) can be caused by the trauma itself (including blunt, nonpenetrating

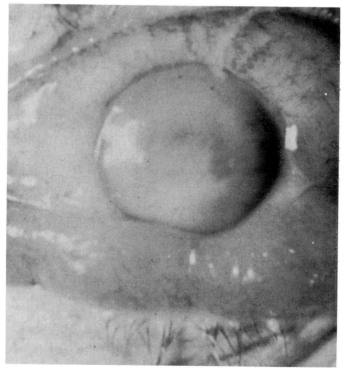

Figure 9–2. Endophthalmitis is signaled by ocular pain, lid edema, chemosis and conjunctival hyperemia, and hypopyon. However, when there has been recent ocular trauma, many of these signs are present even in the absence of true infection. Nonetheless, endophthalmitis must be suspected after any perforating injury. Prophylactic therapy should be initiated immediately, and frequently slit-lamp examinations should be given in the days immediately after repair.

trauma). In addition, sterile copper foreign bodies or sterile lens particles can induce the cardinal signs of inflammation, including a purulent reaction. Nonetheless, the onset of increased pain, decreased clarity of the ocular media, or purulence strongly suggests infection. Whenever an intraocular infection is suspected, prompt diagnostic and therapeutic intervention is justified.

As previously discussed, vitreous cultures are more commonly positive than aqueous cultures in endophthalmitis.[1] Therefore, the vitreous must be sampled to get sufficient material to make a culture diagnosis. Many authorities now agree that the treatment of choice for intraocular infections is intravitreal antibiotics.[4] In practice, the vitreous is tapped through the pars plana, and then antibiotics are injected into the vitreous through the pars plana incision.

Although the optimal antibiotic combination is not known, several suggested regimens are available. An excellent cocktail combines gentamicin, clindamycin, and dexamethasone (Table 9–2). The steroid is added because of the known destructive effect of the inflammation that accompanies the infection. A subconjunctival antibiotic may also be given, although its usefulness is questionable. The patient is then started on intravenous antibiotics, which should be continued for at least seven days.

In cases in which the infection is overwhelming, especially when there is no red reflex, a vitrectomy must often be performed to remove the intraocular abscess and to infuse antibiotics.[5] Antibiotics may be included in the infusion solution (Table 9–3). Although the timing of the vitrectomy is controversial, it seems wise to intervene if the initial therapy of an intravitreal injection fails to result in a stabilization of the inflammatory signs. Should the red reflex continue to deteriorate 12 to 24 hours after the injection, a vitrectomy should be performed.

Table 9–2. ANTIBIOTICS FOR INTRAVITREAL INJECTION IN ENDOPHTHALMITIS

Gentamicin (20 mg/2 ml)	0.40 ml (4.0 mg)
Dexamethasone (10 mg/1 ml)	0.36 ml (3.6 mg)
	0.76 ml
Clindamycin (150 mg/1 ml):	
withdraw from ampule	0.2 ml (30 mg)
and add	1.4 ml sterile saline
	1.6 ml (30 mg/1.6 ml)

Add 0.24 ml of the clindamycin dilution to the gentamicin and dexamethasone to receive final concentration:

Gentamicin 400 mcg ⎫
Dexamethasone 360 mcg ⎬ per 0.1 ml
Clindamycin 450 mcg ⎭

Table 9–3. VITRECTOMY IRRIGATING SOLUTION IN ENDOPHTHALMITIS

Balanced salt solution	500 ml
Sodium bicarbonate 8.4%	13.1 ml
5% Dextrose in water	10 ml
Dexamethasone	8 mg
Gentamicin	4 mg
Clindamycin	4.5 mg

9.3 PROPHYLAXIS OF INFECTIONS

Every physician treating injuries must decide in each case whether or not to prophylactically treat with antibiotics. This decision is especially important in ocular injuries because of the irreparable damage that may be done by an ocular infection.

a. Lid Lacerations

A tetanus immunization history should be obtained from every patient with a lid laceration, and appropriate tetanus prophylaxis must be given. The current recommendations[6] are given in Table 8–2. For most patients, 250 units of tetanus immune globulin given intramuscularly is appropriate. Nearly one fourth of patients with open soft tissue injuries are given inappropriate tetanus treatment.[7]

While clean lid lacerations probably do not require antibiotic prophylaxis, the exact circumstances of the injury are often uncertain. For this reason, many physicians will routinely give a short course of oral antibiotics. Cephalexin has moderately good activity against most of the common pathogens (*Staphylococcus, Pneumococcus, Streptococcus*) and penetrates the periocular tissues very well. Its major disadvantage is the high cost. A cheaper and relatively effective alternative is ampicillin.

b. Orbital Fractures

When the bones of the orbit are fractured, communication with paranasal sinuses often results. Since potentially infected material can then enter the orbit, it is prudent to treat such patients with prophylactic antibiotics. Ampicillin covers the most common sinus pathogen, *Haemophilus influenzae*, and is the best antibiotic in this circumstance. In addition, local or systemic vasoconstrictors (for instance, pseudoephedrine hydrochloride) promote drainage and may be helpful in preventing infection.

c. Penetrating Ocular Injuries

Whether or not the eye retains a foreign body, microorganisms easily enter the eye during penetrating trauma. Disastrous inflammation can occur and may destroy useful vision even if the intraocular contents are sterilized within a few days by antibiotics. Because early diagnosis and therapy are of critical importance if vision is to be salvaged, cultures should be obtained prior to the initiation of prophylactic treatment so that if an infection does occur the potential pathogens may already be identified. Thus, the conjunctiva should be wiped with a culture swab and sent for determination of the conjunctival flora, and if the weapon or object that caused the injury is available it should be cultured. All eyes with perforating injuries should be treated prophylactically with antibiotics to avoid infection.

Systemic therapy is initiated *prior* to surgical repair and should be continued intravenously during the course of the operation and for four days after surgery if no signs of infection occur in that interval. The antibiotics are then discontinued and the patient is watched for any increased inflammation or other signs of early endophthalmitis. If none are present after 24 hours, the patient may be discharged.

The choice of antibiotics is generally empirical but in some cases may be governed by the circumstances of the injury. The general principle is to cover both gram positive and gram negative organisms. An adequate combination is one of methicillin and gentamicin, as these will cover most of the gram positive and gram negative organisms that are likely to cause infection. Penicillin may be added to more fully cover anaerobes if these are likely to be present. Cephalothin or cefazolin provides good coverage of most gram positive organisms and is a good alternative to methicillin and penicillin when given in combination with gentamicin. If *Bacillus cereus* is a suspected pathogen because the perforation involves possibly infected farm implements, gentamicin *and* clindamycin are the only known treatment.[8]

When gentamicin is used, monitoring of the serum creatinine should be done to detect early renal failure and to help in the adjustment of the dosage.

Following completion of the surgical repair, an antibiotic is usually given subconjunctivally. Gentamicin, clindamycin, penicillin, and several other antibiotics have been recommended. In general, gentamicin is an adequate choice.

References

1. Forester RK: Etiology and diagnosis of bacterial postoperative endophthalmitis. Ophthalmology 85:320–326, 1978.
2. Allen HF: Current status of prevention, diagnosis, and management of bacterial corneal ulcers. Ann Ophthalmol 3:235–246, 1971.
3. Baum J, Barza M: Topical vs subconjunctival treatment of bacterial corneal ulcers. Ophthalmology 90:162–168, 1983.

4. Baum J, Peyman GA, Barza M: Intravitreal administration of antibiotics in the treatment of bacterial endophthalmitis. III. Consensus. Surv Ophthalmol 26:204–206, 1982.
5. Peyman GA, Raichand M, Bennett TO: Management of endophthalmitis with pars plana vitrectomy. Br J Ophthalmol 64:472–475, 1980.
6. U. S. Public Health Service, Advisory Committee on Immunization Practices. *Morbidity and Mortality Weekly Report, Supplement.* Vol. 21. No. 25, June 24, 1972, Atlanta, Center for Disease Control.
7. Brand DA, Acampora D, Gottlieb LD, Glancy KE, Frazier WH: Adequacy of antitetanus prophylaxis in six hospital emergency rooms. N Engl J Med 309:636–640, 1983.
8. O'Day BM, Smith RS, Gregg CR, Turnbull PCB, Head WS, Ives JA, Ho PC: The problem of *Bacillus* species infection with special emphasis on the virulence of *Bacillus cereus*. Ophthalmology 88:833–838, 1981.

10

Blunt Injuries of the Globe

A clenched fist or any of a great variety of blunt objects can strike the eye and disrupt its contents. The examiner should take careful stock of the damage (Figure 10–1) resulting from such trauma.

10.1 INJURIES OF THE CONJUNCTIVA

a. Conjunctival Hemorrhage

Conjunctival hemorrhage is the most common accompaniment of ocular trauma (Figures 10–2 and 10–3), but the hemorrhage is, in itself, of no consequence. Spontaneous hemorrhages of the conjunctiva occur in adults of advancing age and in others without apparent reason. Medication does not effectively speed resorption of the hemorrhage, but all traces of hemorrhage should be gone within several weeks. Subconjunctival hemorrhage from orbital bleeding is sometimes so severe that the conjunctiva balloons out between the lids and must be kept lubricated with ointment and/or covered with a plastic film (see Chapter 5) until the swelling subsides and the conjunctiva returns within the lid fissure (Figure 10–4). A cold compress is a good way to minimize swelling in the acute phase.

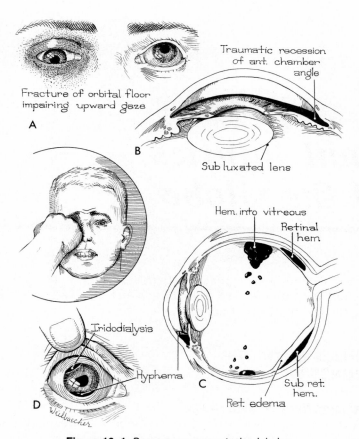

Fracture of orbital floor impairing upward gaze

A

Traumatic recession of ant. chamber angle

B

Subluxated lens

Hem. into vitreous

Retinal hem

C

Sub ret. hem.

Ret. edema

Iridodialysis

Hyphema

D

Figure 10–1. Some common contusion injuries.

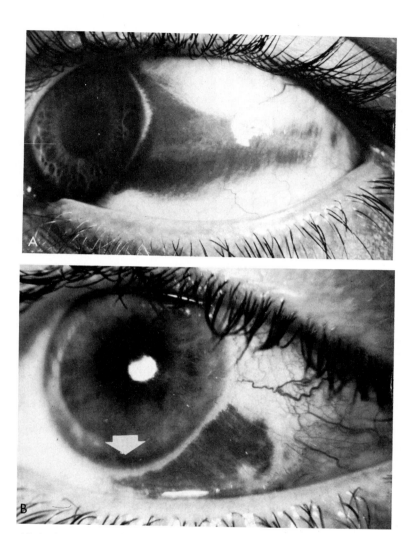

Figure 10–2. (A) Post-traumatic conjunctival hemorrhage without other ocular or orbital damage. (B) Post-traumatic conjunctival hemorrhage from blunt injury with a small hyphema (arrow). In this case, the injury was significant because of the presence of blood in the anterior chamber.

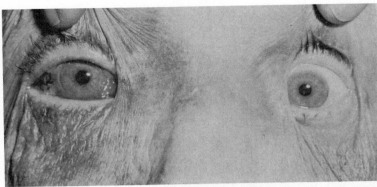

Figure 10–3. Conjunctival and skin hemorrhage resulting from compression injuries to thorax.

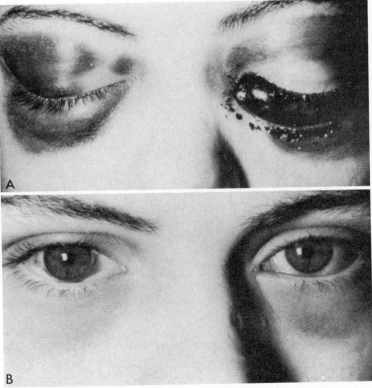

Figure 10–4. (A) A 14-year-old boy with a bleeding disorder sustained blunt trauma to the head resulting in bilateral orbital hemorrhages and hemorrhagic chemosis on the left side. (B) The same patient photographed just ten days later after receiving transfusions of clotting factors. Once the bleeding tendency was corrected, resorption of blood was impressively rapid. During the period of hemorrhagic chemosis, the herniated tissue was kept moist with bland ophthalmic ointment.

b. Chemosis (Conjunctival Edema)

With or without hemorrhage of the conjunctiva, chemosis is often of serious portent (Figure 10–5). Benign causes of conjunctival edema are ultraviolet exposure and various forms of allergic conjunctivitis. Chemosis is also characteristic of endocrine exophthalmos, orbital masses, and trichinosis. *After injury, acute chemosis with pronounced or minimal hemorrhage may be caused by a retained intraorbital foreign body, fracture of the orbit, scleral*

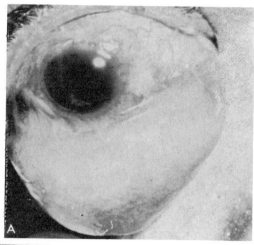

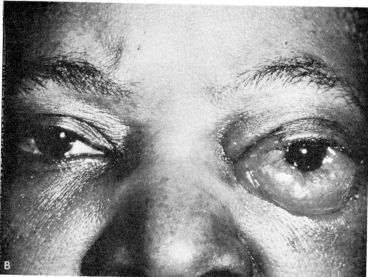

Figure 10–5. Types of chemosis. (A) Chemosis associated with scleral rupture from blunt trauma to the orbit. (B) Chemosis resulting from traumatic carotid-cavernous fistula. There was an orbital bruit and proptosis on the left.

rupture,, carotid-cavernous fistula, or even a tiny, sometimes invisible, scleral perforation. The area of maximum chemosis often is a clue to the location of the scleral rupture or perforation, and this area must be thoroughly examined if the patient is subjected to surgical exploration.

c. Conjunctival Crepitus

Air under the conjunctiva is usually associated with fractures of the lamina papyracea of the ethmoid bone or of the walls of other paranasal sinuses with laceration of the mucosa[1] (see Figure 3–1). Orbital emphysema can result from sneezing, strong nose-blowing, nasal bone or paranasal sinus fractures, and the like. Air in the orbit can reach the lids and, less commonly, the bulbar conjunctiva, where it appears as cystic elevations that are crepitant on palpation.

Compressed air forcefully directed to the eye can also cause conjunctival crepitus as a result of the air stream's tearing a small hole in the conjunctiva.[2]

10.2 HYPHEMA

The term *hyphema* refers to blood within the anterior chamber (Figures 10–6 and 10–7). BB pellets, stones, and fists are notorious causes of hyphemas. Some hyphemas fill the entire anterior chamber, but most are smaller and settle inferiorly, where they can usually be seen with a hand light.

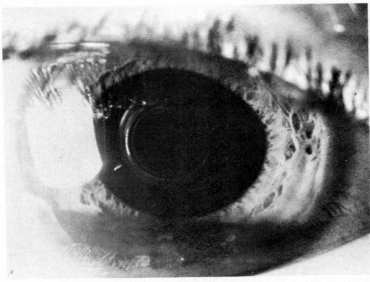

Figure 10–6. A small hyphema resulting from a BB gun injury.

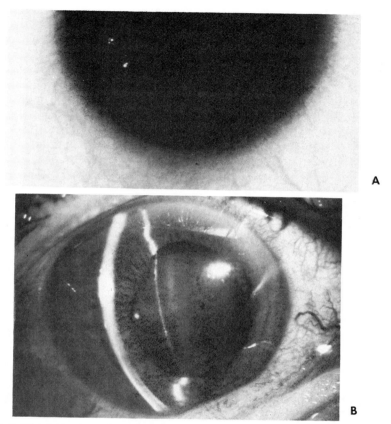

Figure 10–7. (A) total hyphema is present, the intraocular pressure is elevated, there is early blood staining of the cornea (not shown), and there is perilimbal hyperemia. (B) The appearance of an eye after aspiration of a total hyphema. The cornea shows little evidence of blood staining, but there is some distortion of the pupil due to posterior synechias. However, the intraocular pressure is normal, and the lens is clear.

a. Complications

Some approximate statistics may help to put the significance of traumatic hyphema into perspective.[3-9] Between 3 and 33 per cent of hyphemas rebleed. It appears that black patients rebleed at a higher rate than white patients of Scandinavian origin. Of those eyes sustaining initial or secondary *total* hyphema, approximately 25 to 50 per cent will finally have visual acuity of 20/40 or worse, for multiple reasons. Some 5 to 10 per cent of traumatic hyphemas require surgical intervention, using the criteria of most ophthalmic trauma surgeons. About 7 per cent of patients with a history of traumatic hyphema develop glaucoma in later years, and if there has been a large "recession" of the anterior chamber angle (Figure

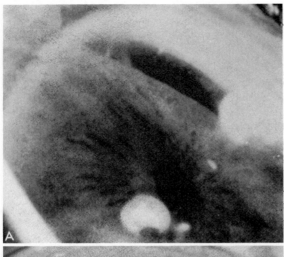

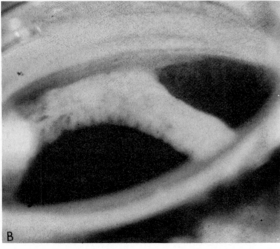

Figure 10–8. Gonioscopic appearance of (A) traumatic recession of the chamber angle and (B) an iridodialysis. The ciliary processes are visible.

10–8), the chances of glaucoma are even greater.[10] Dislocation of the lens and vitreous hemorrhage each occur in approximately 8 per cent of the cases; retinal hemorrhage, though less significant, occurs in over half of the cases.

Rebleeding occurs with greatest frequency between three and five days after initial trauma, and such bleeding almost always begins before the first week has elapsed.[7] The statistical prognosis is immediately worse, and new corneal blood staining and glaucoma are matters of concern.

Somewhat more encouraging than these traditional data are recent reports linking the use of a systemic antifibrinolytic agent, aminocaproic acid, with a sharp decrease in the incidence of rebleeding.[11-13] This drug, in a dose of 50 mg/kg orally every four hours up to a maximum dose of

30 gm/24 hours, minimizes secondary hemorrhage by inhibiting fibrino-
lysis of the clot at the site of injury to the blood vessel.

*The presence of blood in the anterior chamber can be the cause of marked
somnolence through mechanisms that are poorly understood.* Particularly in
children, this "hyphema facies" may be so marked that if the somnolence
is coupled with the history of trauma, an examiner will often recommend
neurologic examination. While the possibility of serious head injury must
always be considered, one should not be surprised if the workup in these
cases is negative.

If the hemorrhage does not resorb promptly, blood pigment may
enter the cornea, where it causes a prolonged tan or rusty-brown staining,
which initially can only be detected by slit-lamp examination. Production
of corneal staining by hematogenous pigment usually requires both a total
hyphema and elevated intraocular pressure. However, in the presence of
diseased corneal endothelium, blood staining occurs more readily. Even
if complete resorption of blood from the anterior chamber later occurs,
corneal translucency or opacity may persist for years. In an infant's eye it
may be the cause of permanent deprivation amblyopia. The extent of
visual loss depends both on the location and intensity of the corneal
staining and on the effect of associated damage to other structures of the
eye. Eventually, the staining clears (Figure 10–9), first peripherally, then
centrally.

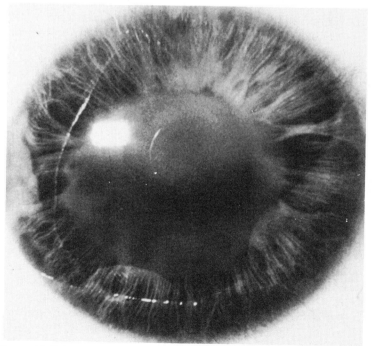

Figure 10–9. Longstanding blood-staining of the cornea, clearing peripherally.

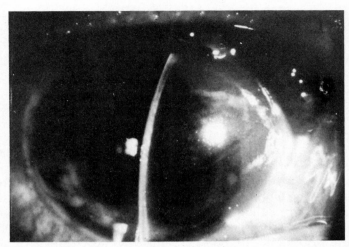

Figure 10–10. Appearance of a total hyphema following trauma. This patient underwent uneventful intracapsular cataract surgery one week prior to injury. On the day of admission, an assailant attacked him, striking a blow to the operated eye.

When the entire anterior chamber is filled with blood it is referred to as a "total hyphema" (Figure 10–10). If the blood does not clear after a few days, the color of the total hyphema changes from red to purple or black (an "eight ball" hyphema). The intraocular pressure is invariably elevated once the hemorrhage changes from red to black, but glaucoma can precede that change. Approximately 25 to 50 per cent of these eyes (for multiple reasons) will have a final visual acuity worse than 20/40.[7, 14] Children under age 6 appear to be most vulnerable.

The prognosis is particularly unfavorable in the case of a total hyphema arising as the result of a secondary hemorrhage. In this circumstance the incidence of good visual recovery is only about 36 per cent.[7]

b. Immediate Management of Hyphemas

The management of hyphemas should be characterized by close attention to the amount of hyphema, the intraocular pressure, and the clarity of the cornea. *Patients should ordinarily be hospitalized and studied at the slit lamp and with applanation tonometry at least daily.* Bilateral patching and absolute bedrest, once the mainstay of hyphema management, have been replaced by less conservative measures as evidence has accumulated in support of this change.[7, 15]

Atropine drops are used to induce cycloplegia for comfort and to dilate the pupil. Dilatation affords an examination of the fundus and prevents pupillary block.

In one prospective study,[6, 7] 137 patients were hospitalized with traumatic hyphema. The results achieved in a group being treated with bedrest, sedation, and bilateral patching were compared with those achieved in a group managed with ambulation *in the hospital*, no sedation, and patching only of the traumatized eye. Patients were assigned alternately to the two treatment groups. Statistical evaluation of admission data showed no significant difference between groups prior to treatment. The duration of grossly visible hyphema and the incidence of elevated intraocular pressure were not different between groups. The duration of elevated intraocular pressure above 24 mm Hg was significantly longer in the bedrest group. Secondary hemorrhage was evaluated by incidence of occurrence, the amount of hyphema before and after rebleed, and the day of occurrence. All comparisons between groups showed no significant differences. Corneal blood staining was encountered in each group in statistically similar numbers. The incidence of recovery of good vision showed no statistically significant difference between groups. Statistical and clinical analyses of these two methods of hyphema therapy indicate, therefore, that bedrest, sedation, and bilateral patching are not significantly more beneficial to *hospitalized* patients than is a regimen of ambulation, no sedation, and patching only of the traumatized eye.

c. *Treatment of Elevated Intraocular Pressure*

The advantages of the *inpatient* management of hyphemas include the careful monitoring and prompt treatment of elevated intraocular pressure. Several drugs are available for use. In most patients, lowering the pressure below 25 mm Hg is sufficient.

Timolol is a safe and effective agent for lowering the intraocular pressure unless the patient has a systemic condition such as asthma or heart block. The dose is one drop every 12 hours.

Acetazolamide is a carbonic anhydrase inhibitor that may be used in adults in a dose of 250 mg every six hours and in children in a dose of 5 mg/kg per dose every six hours. This is the second-line drug started if timolol fails to lower the intraocular pressure below 25 mm Hg.

The use of miotics is controversial because they may result in an exacerbation of the intraocular inflammation. This, in turn, may stymie attempts to lower the intraocular pressure by blocking the outflow mechanism. However, *pilocarpine* is indicated in cases in which surgery is the only alternative. The dose is one drop of the 1 or 2% solution every six hours.

Hyperosmotic agents reduce the intraocular pressure rapidly but transiently. The oral agents are *50% glycerin* and *45% isosorbide*, both administered in a dose of 2 to 4 ml/kg. *Mannitol*, in a 20% solution, is given in a dose of 5 to 10 ml/kg intravenously over a 10- to 20-minute period. Because of the unpredictable absorption of the oral agents and their frequent production of vomiting, mannitol is usually more effective. Caution should be exercised in patients with impaired renal or cardiac function.

d. Indications for Surgery

The proper timing of surgical evacuation of a hyphema is a matter of debate. Uncontrolled secondary glaucoma is the primary concern, and blood staining of the cornea is next in importance. Glaucoma that is difficult to control may occur without a total hyphema. Less frequently, blood staining occurs without a total hyphema.[16] The seriousness of mild blood staining of the cornea may have been overrated in the past (except in very young children), but this sign constitutes another factor in the surgeon's decision, as it is initially difficult to predict whether the staining will become severe. Progression of blood staining from mild to severe can occur over the course of several hours, and the patient must be re-examined frequently if it is elected to delay surgery.

Some surgeons suggest deferring surgery until four days after onset of a total hyphema, because it appears that maximum clot retraction (away from the wall of the eye) without inflammatory organization of fibrosis will take place in that interval.[17]

The surgeon's decision as to when and how to operate depends on a thorough knowledge of the injured eye gained from daily slit-lamp examinations and frequent pressure determinations. If the lens is subluxated, surgery for the hyphema is more likely to be deferred, as there is a high chance of disturbing the vitreous. If a bleeding site has been observed or if there is an iridodialysis (the presumed bleeding site), a constructive approach to the prevention of further rebleeding from the dialysis site can be included with surgery for the hyphema itself (see below).

Many total hyphemas clear spontaneously. If the intraocular pressure is normal and the cornea is clear, then there is no justification for surgical intervention. On the other hand, surgical intervention should be performed to *prevent* the major complications of hyphema and induced ocular hypertension: blood staining of the cornea, optic atrophy, and peripheral anterior synechias.

Data from a prospective clinical trial are available to assist the surgeon in making the decision about when surgery is indicated[7] (Table 10–1). Optic nerve damage may be anticipated with intraocular pressures of approximately 50 mm Hg or more for at least five days (or 35 mm Hg for at least seven days). Blood staining of the cornea may be anticipated with increasing frequency in cases of total hyphema when intraocular pressures of 25 mm Hg or more are present for at least six days. Peripheral anterior synechias in unoperated eyes may be anticipated with hyphemas lasting

Table 10–1. GUIDELINES FOR SURGICAL INTERVENTION IN HYPHEMAS

1. To prevent optic atrophy:
    a. Operate **before** the intraocular pressure has **averaged** > *50 mm Hg for five days.*
    b. Operate **before** the intraocular pressure has **averaged** > *35 mm Hg for seven days.*
2. To prevent corneal blood staining:
    a. Operate **before** the intraocular pressure has **averaged** > *25 mm Hg for six days.*
    b. Operate when there is any indication of *early blood staining.*
3. To prevent peripheral anterior synechiae:
    a. Operate **before** *a total hyphema persists for five days.*
    b. Operate **before** *a diffuse hyphema persists for nine days.*
4. Operate when there is persistent elevated intraocular pressure from pupillary block.

nine days or more. Because these figures represent pressures and dura-
tions when complications may be expected, it is recommended that
surgical intervention be carried out *prior* to reaching these limits. Therefore, surgical removal of the blood may be considered whenever any of
these conditions is anticipated or as soon as *microscopic* corneal blood
staining is seen.[6]

e. Surgical Techniques

Opinions on the several approaches to the surgical management of
traumatic hyphema continue to spark controversy.[6] It seems appropriate
to divide the techniques into several groups.

Simple Paracentesis. During the first four days, most hyphemas will
be diffuse and unclotted. It is often possible to permanently lower the
intraocular pressure by performing a simple paracentesis. After taking
precautions to prevent infection (careful prepping and draping), topical
or local anesthetics are used for analgesia. The globe is firmly grasped
either 180 degrees from the intended entry site or directly at that site. A
25- or 27-gauge tuberculin syringe is used. The plunger is removed from
the barrel, and the needle is slowly advanced through clear cornea,
keeping it parallel to the iris at all times. For safety, the eye should be
entered tangentially, so that the needle's tip will be positioned over the
iris instead of the lens when it is in the anterior chamber. Once the bevel
of the needle is within the anterior chamber, it is tilted up toward the
dome of the cornea, and aqueous is allowed to enter the barrel of the
syringe until the eye begins to collapse. The needle is then quickly pulled
from the eye. The intraocular pressure should be rechecked in two hours
to determine whether the procedure was effective.

Aspiration Techniques. A firm, retracted clot usually has developed
four days after the onset of a *total* hyphema. Until the end of this interval
(and sometimes even after this interval), cases of total hyphema with
severe, uncontrollable glaucoma or early signs of blood staining can be
managed by the simple aspiration technique. Although a two-needle

technique has traditionally been used, the development of double-barreled needles for use in manual extracapsular cataract surgery has made this procedure much safer than previously. A beveled incision is made through the superior limbus and the instrument introduced into the anterior chamber under visualization with the operating microscope. The tip must be visualized at all times during the procedure for the protection of the corneal endothelium and the lens capsule. The infusion port is connected to a bottle of irrigating solution, and the bottle is maintained at a level approximately 50 cm above the operative field. This will keep the intraocular pressure sufficiently high to tamponade the fragile blood vessels on the face of the ciliary body. If one of the ports is larger than the other, the larger port must be used for the infusion and the smaller for the aspiration. Such an arrangement will prevent the anterior chamber from shallowing during aspiration. Gentle suction is applied to remove free red blood cells, and the infusion port may be moved around in the anterior chamber to create a swirling effect, which will result in removal of more blood. *There is no need to remove all traces of blood.* The bottle should be slowly lowered to 25 cm above the field at the end of the procedure and a search made for any rebleeding. If there is persistent hemorrhage, the bottle is again raised and the hyphema aspirated. A large air bubble may be left in the eye to tamponade the bleeding vessel. The instrument is removed from the eye, and a single 9-0 or 10-0 nylon suture may be placed in the wound to achieve a watertight seal.

Large Incision Technique. Usually by the fourth day, a clot filling the anterior chamber has become firm and retracted, and irrigation is sometimes inadequate to remove it. If surgical intervention is deemed necessary at this point, the clot should be removed through a large incision with a limbus-based flap and entrance into the anterior chamber comparable to that used in intracapsular cataract extraction.[14] Without introducing instruments into the anterior chamber, the surgeon applies gentle manual pressure at the 6-o'clock position of the limbus to express the clot. (A cryoprobe should not be used to assist in delivering the clot, as it can adhere to the iris and even to the lens, causing severe damage.) Preplaced sutures are then tightened, tied, and cut, and the conjunctival flap is separately closed. The main points in this method of surgical intervention are the following: The incision must be a large one, preferably 120 to 160 degrees. Instruments should not be placed into the anterior chamber to avoid inadvertent iridodialysis, iridectomy, or lens trauma.

The large solid clot may actually deliver itself when the anterior chamber is opened, and the surgeon may be alarmed at the size and color, possibly thinking that the entire uveal tract is prolapsing. Rebleeding may result from overly vigorous attempts at rinsing the excess blood from the anterior chamber. Rarely, a bleeding vessel is visible enough to be treated directly. Cautery of the vessel itself can be effective, with surprisingly little postoperative iritis.

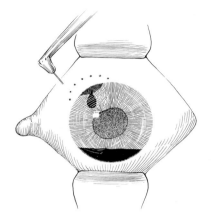

Figure 10–11. Recurrent hyphema. Occasionally a bleeding site can be identified at the time of hyphema recurrence. Such cases are best treated by diathermy to the ciliary body and iris root in the area from which the bleeding has arisen.

Special Techniques. With the advent of the automated irrigation/aspiration machines for cataract surgery and the automated vitreous suction/cutters for vitrectomy surgery, the removal of dense clots through a small incision is possible. Unfortunately, the smaller models of these instruments have small aspiration ports, which often cannot aspirate large clots, and use of the larger instruments with sufficiently large aspiration ports may result in inadvertent injury to the lens or cornea unless extraordinary care is taken to avoid these structures.

Some reports indicate that aspiration of a hyphema is more readily accomplished by the use of intracameral fibrinolytic agents (urokinase, fibrinolysin),[18] but conclusions regarding the use of these agents have not been uniform.

Direct Treatment of the Bleeding Site; Iridodialysis Repair. When repeated bleeding has occurred from a single site or when multiple rebleeds occur in an eye with iridodialysis, surgical intervention should be accompanied by an effort to cauterize the bleeding site with transscleral diathermy[19] (Figure 10–11). A 2.5-mm diathermy pin is used for multiple punctures 2 to 4 mm from the limbus sufficient in number to cause scarring of the ciliary body in the region, giving rise to the hemorrhage.

f. Sickle Cell Hemoglobinopathy and Hyphema

Patients with sickle cell hemoglobinopathies, including the otherwise "benign" sickle cell trait, are at increased risk for many of the complications of traumatic hyphemas.[20] Red blood cells become sickled in the "hostile" environment of the anterior chamber with its low pH and relative hypoxia as compared with the bloodstream. Cells in the sickle configuration cannot egress through the outflow channels of the eye, and the intraocular pressure may be very high even with a microscopic hyphema. This high pressure, in turn, impedes blood flow through the vascular supply of the optic nerve and retina, and optic atrophy or central retinal artery occlusion may occur. Slowed blood flow through these vessels may also result in increased sickling of the "sludged" red blood cells. The blood supply of the anterior segment may also be impeded, with resultant further hypoxia in the anterior chamber and further sickling. Thus, a vicious circle is set up, with ever more sickling, more ischemia, more sickling, and so on.[21]

Medical Treatment. The guidelines for treatment of patients with uncomplicated cases are the same as those for patients with normal hemoglobin. Elevated intraocular pressure is treated with the same drugs as stated previously with two exceptions. Methazolamide is used instead of acetazolamide as a carbonic anhydrase inhibitor because it is said to have less of a pH lowering effect in the anterior chamber. Hyperosmotic agents are given only once in any 24-hour period to avoid a systemic hyperviscosity, which could result in increased sickling in the small vessels supplying the optic nerve head.

Surgical Indications. A retrospective study has found that medical therapy generally results in adequate control of the intraocular pressure. However, in patients in whom the intraocular pressure remains greater than 24 mm Hg for longer than 24 hours despite medical therapy, it is not possible to lower the pressure adequately, no matter how long the medical therapy is continued.[20] As Goldberg has stated that the visual prognosis may be worse if the intraocular pressure is allowed to remain above 24 mm Hg for longer than 24 hours,[21] it is recommended that some form of surgical therapy be carried out before 24 hours of elevated intraocular pressure have elapsed. At the time of publication a multicenter national trial sponsored by the National Institutes of Health is under way to evaluate the necessity of this aggressive approach.

10.3 INJURIES OF THE ANTERIOR UVEA

a. Traumatic Iritis

A mild inflammation of the iris and ciliary body may follow almost any trauma to the eye. The intraocular pressure is lower than normal in the early post-traumatic period, and the aqueous humor contains cells and fibrin. A cycloplegic agent is used to make the patient comfortable. In severe cases, topical steroids may be used, but development of posterior synechia is uncommon when no hyphema is present.

b. Traumatic Mydriasis and Miosis

More severe blows can, in addition, be accompanied by dilatation or constriction of the pupil, *traumatic mydriasis,* or miosis that may persist for several days or considerably longer. The pupil reacts minimally; it is often slightly irregular. Hard blows to the eye commonly produce a rupture of the iris sphincter (Figure 10–12) and permanent deformity of the pupil.

c. Traumatic Recession of the Anterior Chamber Angle

Blunt trauma to the eye frequently causes unilateral glaucoma that may develop months or years after the injury. In many of these cases, the blow has caused a cleft or recession in the tissues of the anterior chamber angle, the most important site of aqueous drainage from the eye (see Figure 10–8). Depending on the series reported, 20 to 100 per cent of eyes sustaining traumatic hyphema have chamber angle recession,[10, 22-24] thereby predisposing to glaucoma.

Followup studies on eyes with a history of traumatic hyphema indicate that there is approximately a 7 per cent incidence of late onset of glaucoma. Thus, all patients who have had hyphema should remain under an ophthalmologist's care. Apparently, the greater the traumatic recession of the angle (in terms of circumferential extent), the greater the chance of

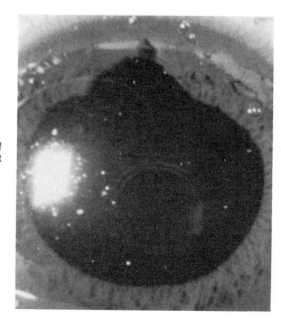

Figure 10–12. Traumatic rupture of the iris sphincter resulting from blunt trauma to the eye.

developing glaucoma in subsequent months or years. This seems especially true when the angle damage is more than 180 degrees.[25]

10.4 INJURIES OF THE LENS

a. Subluxation and Dislocation of the Lens

Blunt trauma to the globe can break the zonular fibers that encircle the lens radially and anchor it to the ciliary body. When more than 25 per cent of the fibers are broken, the lens is said to be *subluxated*, and it is no longer held securely against the posterior surface of the iris. When all of the fibers are broken, the lens is *dislocated* and may fall posteriorly into the vitreous cavity or may move anteriorly into the pupillary space or anterior chamber. Trembling of the iris (iridodonesis) is frequently observed with the hand-held flashlight or slit lamp while the patient moves the eye quickly back and forth.

Certain diseases predispose to weakening of the zonular fibers, after which relatively minor trauma may lead to subluxation or dislocation; Marfan's syndrome, syphilis, Marchesani's syndrome,[26] and hemocystinuria are classic examples.

b. Indications for Surgery

Emergency surgery for dislocation of the lens is usually required only when the lens is entirely within the anterior chamber or is incarcerated in the pupil, causing glaucoma. Either condition can result in an acute rise in intraocular pressure, necessitating prompt action. In addition, if the lens is entirely in the anterior chamber, permanent damage to the corneal endothelium may occur unless the lens is removed within several hours.

Location of the lens within the anterior chamber impedes or prevents aqueous from gaining access to the outflow channels of the eye, and elevated intraocular pressure often results. If a lens occludes the pupillary space by being incarcerated within it, continued production of aqueous into the posterior chamber pushes the peripheral iris anteriorly, thereby obstructing the outflow channel. This sequence of events produces *pupillary block glaucoma*. When the zonule is broken and the lens is subluxated, vitreous may herniate through the zonular defect into the pupil (Figure 10–13) and may also cause pupillary block glaucoma.

Intravitreal dislocation of the lens is a serious complication of ocular trauma but never requires emergency lens extraction. If the capsule is intact, there is very little risk of acute glaucoma. These patients are usually managed by waiting for the inflammation to subside and then fitting the patient with a contact lens if the visual axis is clear.

Figure 10–13. Traumatic rupture of the zonules with herniation of vitreous through the pupillary space. It is important to recognize the presence of vitreous in the anterior chamber prior to removal of a cataractous lens. The high risk of vitreous extrusion through the surgical incision can then be minimized by avoiding preoperative massage of the eye, by administering systemic hyperosmotic agents, or by aspirating liquid vitreous through a needle introduced through the pars plana. Aspiration creates a risk that the lens will move posteriorly into the vitreous, making it inaccessible at the time of surgery.

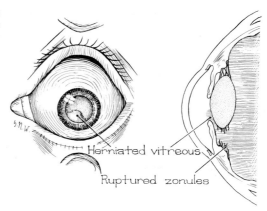

Herniated vitreous

Ruptured zonules

c. Management by Surgery

Surgical management of some types of dislocated lenses is usually thought to be attended by considerable hazards.[27, 28] In one series there was a 41 per cent incidence of vitreous loss at the time of lens extraction.[28] One third of these operated eyes subsequently became blind, and lens extraction cured glaucoma in only one third. Thus, until recently, the prognosis for these eyes has been quite poor.

Several advances in recent years have improved the outlook for eyes with lens injuries. Argon or Neodymium/YAG lasers can be used to make iridotomies and break pupillary block. Automated irrigation/aspiration instruments have become widely available to aspirate subluxated lenses. Automated vitreous suction/cutters have been developed that can be used to remove the lens as well as manage the vitreous.

When surgery on an anteriorly located or subluxated lens is *necessary*, three basic types of surgical intervention should be considered, and *the choice must be based on the experience of the surgeon* and the availability of certain instrumentation.

Intracapsular Subluxated Lens Extraction. Individuals of age 40 or more should have intracapsular lens extraction. After intravenous mannitol has been started, a limbus-based conjunctival flap is made and a conventional intracapsular lens extraction is initiated. Preplaced sutures and a peripheral or sector iridectomy are routine. On entering the anterior chamber, no vitrectomy should be done, for this might allow the lens to sink out of sight. A cryoprobe at room temperature is introduced through the wound and touched to the surface of the lens (through overlying vitreous if necessary); then freezing is started. When the ice ball is formed, the lens is delivered through the wound. Vitreous traction must be minimized, and the assistant may have to cut strands of vitreous from the back of the lens as it is removed from the eye. The surgeon then proceeds with an anterior vitrectomy, if necessary, using cellulose sponges or a vitrectomy instrument. Vitreous disturbance is not invariable, but when it occurs, the anterior chamber should be left free of vitreous. Only then should the incision be closed.

As an alternative, a sclerotomy may be made at the beginning of the procedure, prior to entering the anterior chamber, and once the lens is removed and the wound closed, a pars plana vitrectomy may be done (see below).

Lens Aspiration. If the lens is trapped in the anterior chamber without vitreous present or if it is subluxated but visible within the pupillary space, simple aspiration of the lens is possible, using one of several similar methods.[29-31] In brief, a young patient's subluxated lens can be fixed in position with one needle while being aspirated from within its capsule with another. A previously intact vitreous face will remain intact in many cases. If an admixture of vitreous and lens material develops, the surgeon can resort to a vitrectomy procedure, either through the limbal incision or through an incision 2 to 3 mm posterior to the limbus.

Pars Plana Lensectomy and Vitrectomy. The technique of pars plana surgery using the Peyman Vitreophage has been described elsewhere.[32] Briefly, the conjunctiva is dissected to expose an area of sclera 3 to 5 mm posterior to the limbus. A sclerotomy is prepared 3 mm from the limbus, which is 3.5 mm long running parallel to the limbus. Light cautery is applied to the underlying uvea, and a 5-0 Vicryl suture is preplaced in a mattress fashion in the sclerotomy. A sharp knife is used to enter the vitreous and lens through the ciliary body, and the Vitreophage is then carefully placed perpendicularly into the vitreous and finally into the lens. After temporarily tying the suture to provide a closed system, the lens is suctioned and cut and an anterior vitrectomy is done. In experienced hands, a floating contact lens can be placed on the cornea to visualize the posterior segment, enabling the surgeon to do a complete vitrectomy. The Vitreophage is then pulled from the eye and the suture is simultaneously tied. If the intraocular pressure is low, irrigation fluid is used to re-form the eye.

d. Contusion Cataract

Even without detectable damage to the lens capsule, contusion injuries can lead to secondary cataract (Figure 10–14). As a result of forceful impact of the iris against the anterior surface of the lens, a Vossius ring can be produced (Figure 10–15). This circle of iris pigment on the lens is rarely noticed until the pupil is dilated. It has no clinical significance other than as a diagnostic sign of previous blunt trauma. Anterior cortical lens vacuoles, anterior nodular plaques, posterior cortical changes, wedge-shaped and generalized opacities, and intumescence may ensue.

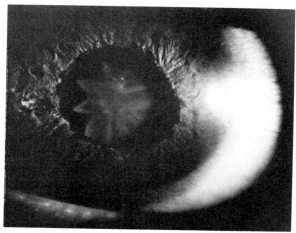

Figure 10–14. Traumatic cataract secondary to blunt injury. Despite the lens opacity, the patient retained a visual acuity of 20/40.

10.5 SCLERAL RUPTURE

A blow to the eye sometimes produces rupture of the globe; the conjunctiva may remain intact. The most common rupture sites are in a circumferential arc parallel to the corneal limbus (see Figure 8–3) opposite the impact site, at the insertion of the rectus muscles on the globe, and at the equator of the eyeball. The most common quadrant is supranasal, near

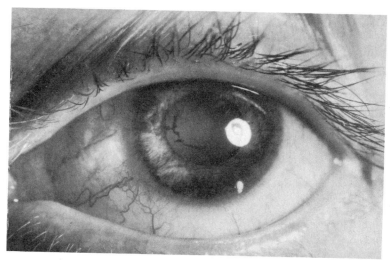

Figure 10–15. An eye with history of blunt trauma demonstrating faint Vossius ring on the anterior lens capsule.

the limbus,[33] but *a scleral rupture can be present without being visible to the examiner.*

Rupture is suspected when the anterior chamber is filled with blood, the eye is soft, and there is marked hemorrhagic chemosis of the conjunctiva out of proportion to the apparent injury. In addition, the chemosis may be localized to one quadrant, overlying the rupture. Occasionally, the intraocular pressure may be normal or even elevated.[33] Duction of the globe may be reduced toward the quadrant harboring the rupture. The anterior chamber may be abnormally deep. Some eyes with rupture near the limbus have total extraocular luxation of the lens to a subconjunctival position (see Figure 8–4).

The prognosis for vision is reduced when the lens is involved. In addition, the more posterior and longer the rupture, the worse the prognosis.[34, 35] An attempt to repair the eye is almost always justified, particularly if it has been the patient's better eye. Surgical principles are the same as those for repair of scleral laceration (see Chapter 8).

10.6 VITREOUS HEMORRHAGE

Hemorrhage into the vitreous from trauma is usually caused by damage to a retinal, ciliary-body, or choroidal vessel. Eyes with pathologically altered blood vessels are particularly vulnerable; diabetes, sickle cell diseases, and other disorders with retinal neovascularization predispose to hemorrhage. Loss of vision may be sudden and profound, and the site of pathology may be obscured from the examiner's view.

Since retinal tears are a major cause of vitreous hemorrhage, a careful search for a retinal detachment must be made in all cases of vitreous hemorrhage. In addition, the possibility of a rupture of the sclera must be kept in mind, and the inability to see the entire fundus may be a major factor in a decision to conduct a surgical exploration for a rupture site.

a. Diagnosis

The indirect ophthalmoscope is the most useful tool for examining patients with vitreous hemorrhage. With its bright illumination, the examiner may be able to detect the presence of a posterior vitreous detachment, a retinal tear or detachment, or a choroidal rupture. *Every patient with blunt trauma to the globe should have a dilated fundus examination at the initial visit.* The first examiner may be the only physician to see fundus details for quite some time, as additional vitreous hemorrhage may obscure an adequate view.

The slit lamp biomicroscope may be helpful when focal areas of preretinal hemorrhage require a close examination to find their cause. A variety of contact lenses are available for this purpose.

When the view of the fundus is obscured by diffuse blood, an ultrasound examination is necessary to determine the status of the retina. Both A-scan and B-scan ultrasonography are useful in diagnosing retinal detachments and in locating intraocular foreign bodies.[36]

Computerized tomography has become more useful as experience with the technique and its interpretation has accumulated. The diagnosis of hemorrhagic choroidal detachment, retinal detachment, scleral rupture, intraocular foreign bodies, and optic nerve sequelae of blunt trauma can be greatly aided by high-quality scans. Preferably, the "cuts" should be 2 mm or less in thickness.

b. Treatment

The treatment of vitreous hemorrhage is initially expectant; most vitreous hemorrhages eventually resorb, and the underlying pathology can then be detected and sometimes treated. A trial of bed rest for several days with binocular occlusion is useful. The head of the bed is constantly elevated to reduce the pressure within the intraocular blood vessels and to allow the effect of gravity to cause settling of intravitreal blood inferior to the visual axis. This occurs most often in older patients and in patients whose vitreous is liquefied. If settling of the vitreous blood occurs, continuation of this therapy is indicated until improvement ceases. If no consolidation of the blood is noted, it may be weeks or months before clearing occurs; it is therefore best to allow the patient to resume his normal routine if it does not involve vigorous physical activity. The status of the retina can be monitored from time to time by ultrasonography.

Unresorbed old vitreous hemorrhage in an eye otherwise considered to be functional can be removed with notable success by pars plana vitrectomy. The presence of a posterior vitreous detachment (diagnosed preoperatively by ultrasound) makes this surgery much easier, as most of the vitreous can then be easily removed without approaching the retinal surface. Many times, when the posterior hyaloid is penetrated by the vitreous cutter, thick preretinal blood is encountered that must be patiently irrigated and suctioned until it no longer obscures the view of the instruments. A fiberoptic light inserted through a separate pars plana incision greatly facilitates these operations.

Vitrectomy for vitreous hemorrhage, in the absence of a retinal detachment, is elective surgery and should be performed only after the blood has been given sufficient time to resorb spontaneously; this is often six months or longer.

10.7 RETINAL BREAKS AND DETACHMENTS

Of all retinal detachments, trauma has probably played a primary role in only 15 per cent.[37] Retinal detachments from ocular trauma are usually late sequelae of the original injury; about 80 per cent occur within two years of the responsible trauma.[38] On the other hand, when a retinal break develops as a result of trauma, the chance of the retina detaching within several weeks is high enough that such a break should be closed at the earliest possible time. When the retina detaches soon after contusion of the eye, the detachment may also be due to antecedent vitreoretinal pathology, which, after potentiation by blunt trauma, leads to retinal tears and detachment.

a. Diagnosis

Suspicion is an important tool in the diagnosis of retinal detachment. A retinal break is suspected when there is a history of a shower of black specks, "light flashes," and a curtainlike defect in the peripheral field of vision. Examination with an ophthalmoscope often reveals a billow of grayish retina that shifts with changes in the patient's eye position. Typical traumatic retinal detachments are usually associated with far peripheral retinal tears that cannot be seen with a hand ophthalmoscope. A common type of retinal break seen in these detachments is a dialysis (disinsertion of the retina) at the posterior border of the vitreous base, especially in the superonasal but also in the inferotemporal quadrant of the eye.[39] Detachment from a dialysis is usually a late occurrence, and a patient may have even forgotten the original traumatic event. Avulsion of the vitreous base has been considered to be pathognomonic of traumatic retinal detachment,[38] but other clues such as iris sphincter tears and angle recession may alert the surgeon to a traumatic etiology.

In patients with dense vitreous hemorrhage, ultrasound techniques are invaluable in aiding in the diagnosis of a retinal detachment. A highly reflective posterior echo, especially if attached at the disc, is highly suggestive of a detachment.

b. Treatment

New retinal breaks caused by trauma should be closed as soon as possible. This can be accomplished using either photocoagulation or cryocoagulation, depending on the location and the size of the break, the availability of equipment, and the experience and preference of the surgeon.

When a retinal detachment is present, especially if a dialysis is present or if there is vitreous traction on the break, a scleral buckling procedure should be done as soon as it is feasible, especially if the macula is threatened or has only recently become detached. When a giant tear of 90 to 180 degrees occurs, the case should be handled as an emergency to prevent further extension that would make the surgical prognosis much less favorable.

Since vitreous hemorrhage damages the vitreous structure and can lead to formation of vitreous bands that pull on the retina, it is easy to understand why retinal tears and retinal detachment can be late sequelae of traumatic vitreous hemorrhage. But contusion injury alone, without hemorrhage into the vitreous, may also lead to the late occurrence of retinal detachment. These factors are very difficult to appraise, but they have visual and medicolegal implications of such importance that they constitute further reasons for extensive examination of the peripheral retina of every traumatized eye as soon as indirect ophthalmoscopy and scleral depression are possible.[40]

10.8 TRAUMATIC CHORIORETINAL DISORDERS

Either direct blows to the eye or contrecoup trauma from blows to the back of the head can produce retinal edema with or without reduction in vision, depending on the location. If the examiner is uncertain as to whether there is retinal edema, comparison with the other eye is helpful. Retinal edema, such as Berlin's edema (see below), appears as a whitish, geographic, cloudy discoloration against the homogeneous red-orange background of the normal ocular fundus.

A short time after concussion injury to the eye, large subretinal hemorrhages may be found; these are often accompanied by intraretinal and superficial retinal hemorrhages, which appear as brighter red than the grayish-blue or purple of deep (subretinal or pigment epithelial) hemorrhages. Preretinal (subhyaloid) hemorrhages may also occur and layer in a "boat-shaped" pattern.

Vision is not necessarily affected unless macular hemorrhage or macular edema occurs or unless, in the ensuing days, hard retinal exudates form in a star configuration at the macula. In these last two circumstances the prognosis for macular function is poor.

Little can be done to treat traumatic fundus lesions, with the possible exception of retinal artery occlusion. Nevertheless, an understanding of the following distinct entities may help in prognostication for the patient.

a. Berlin's Edema (Commotio Retinae, Concussion Edema)

Retinal edema is commonplace after direct blows to the eye. When severe, it can affect the entire posterior pole and may simulate a central retinal artery occlusion,[37] producing a "pseudo-cherry red spot" (Figure 10–16). The vision is reduced, and late pigmentary macular changes may ensue. The prognosis for central acuity is guarded, and a macular cyst or hole may develop, as it may with other concussion retinopathies[41] (Figures

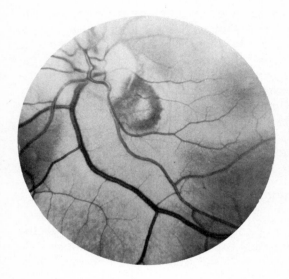

Figure 10–16. Berlin's edema of the posterior pole following blunt injury. Note that the macular appearance is that of a "pseudo-cherry red spot." The visual acuity returned to 20/20 one month following the accident.

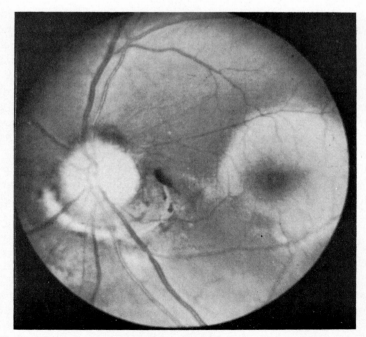

Figure 10–17. Edema, hemorrhages, and a choroidal rupture surround the optic nervehead. There is also edema of the macula (Berlin's edema) in this eye, which has sustained blunt trauma.

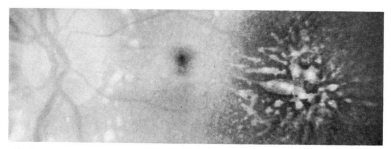

Figure 10–18. The fundus appearance in the eye of a 7-year-old boy who received blunt trauma to the occiput from a medicine ball. Hard exudates are seen in the macular and peripapillary areas.

10–17 and 10–18). The etiology of this condition remains controversial. Most authorities believe that, contrary to the name, there is no actual retinal edema. It is postulated that a derangement of the photoreceptors occurs, contributing to the poor vision and deep retinal whitening seen with Berlin's edema. Others believe that the discrete white lesions are areas of choroidal lobular ischemia. While there is no evidence for this theory, the geographic, circumscribed, and evanescent nature of the areas supports this hypothesis.

b. Retinal, Subretinal, and Preretinal Hemorrhages

Retinal, preretinal, and subretinal hemorrhages are also common after concussion injury. They are generally of minimal significance, although macular dysfunction of a permanent nature may occur if the hemorrhage involves that region. Exudates and edema may accompany the retinal hemorrhage, indicating at least temporary impairment of small vessel function.

c. Rupture of the Choroid

Severe concussion injury to the globe can produce a rupture of the choroid that at the time of the initial examination appears only as a large fundus hemorrhage at the posterior pole of the eye, occasionally breaking through into the vitreous (Figure 10–19). Late clearing of this hemorrhage permits view of a curvilinear yellow-white scar, which may transect the macula and cause permanent impairment of vision. Neovascularization of choroidal ruptures may also occur, and can, months and years later, lead to transudation, hemorrhage, and macular detachment.[42]

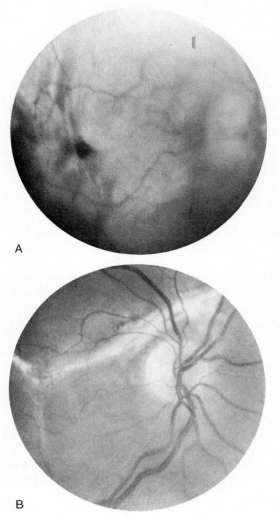

A

B

Figure 10–19. Choroidal rupture following blunt injury. (A) This patient was hit in the right eye with a metal garbage can. There was immediate loss of vision. Blood can be seen under the retinal pigment epithelium and is also coming through the foveal pit into the vitreous. (B) Three months following the injury, curvilinear choroidal ruptures can be observed in the posterior pole, extending through the fovea. The visual acuity was finger counting.

d. Chorioretinitis Sclopetaria

A concussive, nonpenetrating injury caused by an orbital missile (such as a gunshot) that is characterized by choroidal *and* retinal rupturing[43] is called chorioretinitis sclopetaria. With this condition the sclera usually remains intact. In the early stages, there is extensive hemorrhage (usually including the vitreous); when the hemorrhage clears, fibrosis and retinal destruction are observed (Figure 10–20). The vision is invariably poor. However, the retina rarely detaches, presumably because it is incorporated by fibrosis into the wall of the eye.

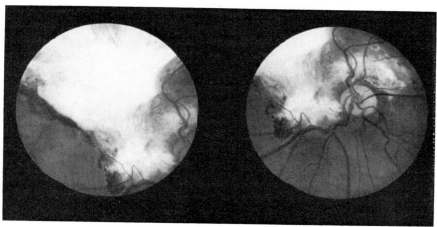

A

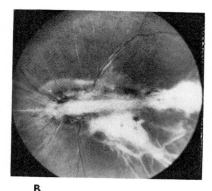

B

Figure 10–20. (A) Retinitis sclopetaria. The chorioretinal scarring and optic atrophy in this eye are the result of a bullet wound. Fired at close range, the bullet traversed the posterior orbit and entered the contralateral orbit, where it destroyed the globe and passed through the lateral orbital wall. Patient retains 10/400 vision in the remaining eye and makes effective use of low-vision aids. (B) A late view of a traumatic avulsion of the optic nerve. Although the eye is normal in external appearance, there is no light perception.

e. Fat Emboli

Fractures of the long bones can produce fatty emboli that may escape into the venous circulation, circumnavigate the pulmonary circulation, gain access to the heart, and then reach the retinal vasculature.[44] In the eye, these emboli appear as hard yellow-white retinal exudates. They may be accompanied by edema and flame-shaped hemorrhages. The lesions are larger than cholesterol emboli of carotid artery origin and are not as refractile. They should be distinguished from drusen, cotton-wool patches, and talc or cornstarch emboli reported in drug abusers.[45] The retinal lesions themselves have little significance, although a central retinal artery occlusion is a theoretical possibility. Emboli also cause significant symptoms when they lodge in the lungs and brain.

f. Ocular Sequelae of Compression Injuries

The condition known as *Purtscher's retinopathy* is caused by sudden thoracic compression (as in crush injuries). The ocular findings are those associated with fat emboli (hard yellow-white exudates, arterial spasm, striate and preretinal hemorrhages, localized edema, and fluffy transudates.[37, 46, 47] Prognosis for good vision is favorable, as in the case of fat emboli. Purtscher's syndrome is not compounded by cerebral and pulmonary symptoms such as those caused by fat embolization.

Traumatic asphyxia is a syndrome characterized by blue discoloration of the face, neck, and upper chest. Like Purtscher's retinopathy, traumatic asphyxia results from severe compression of the thorax.[48] The eyelids are blue, the conjunctiva is hemorrhagic, and proptosis may occur. The retina is usually normal (unlike that in Purtscher's syndrome), but edema, hemorrhages, cotton-wool spots, and papilledema have been described. The visual prognosis is excellent, and the status of ocular structures will return to normal if the case is not fatal.

References

1. Byrnes VA: Elevated intravascular pressure as an etiologic mechanism in the production of eye injuries. Trans Am Ophthalmol Soc 57:473–538, 1959.
2. Walsh MA: Orbitopalpebral emphysema and traumatic uveitis from compressed air injury. Arch Ophthalmol 87:228–229, 1972.
3. Coles WH: Traumatic hyphema: an analysis of 235 cases. South Med J 61:813–816, 1968.
4. Edwards WC, Layden WE: Monocular versus binocular patching in traumatic hyphema. Am J Ophthalmol 76:359–362, 1973.
5. Havener WH: Ocular Pharmacology. (Third Edition). St. Louis, C. V. Mosby Co, 1974.
6. Read J, Goldberg MF: Blunt ocular trauma and hyphema. Int Ophthalmol Clin 14:57–95, 1974.
7. Read J, Goldberg MF: Comparison of medical treatment of traumatic hyphema. Trans Am Acad Ophthalmol Otolaryngol 78:OP799–OP815, 1974.
8. Spaeth GL, Levy PM: Traumatic hyphema: its clinical characteristics and failure of estrogens to alter its course: a double blind study. Am J Ophthalmol 62:1098–1106, 1966.
9. Uusitalo RJ, Saari MS, Aine E, Saari KM: Tranexamic acid in the prevention of secondary haemorrhage after traumatic hyphaema. Acta Ophthalmol 59:539–545, 1981.
10. Blanton FM: Anterior chamber angle recession and secondary glaucoma: a study of the after effects of traumatic hyphemas. Arch Ophthalmol 72:39–43, 1964.
11. Crouch ER, Frenkel M: Aminocaproic acid in the treatment of traumatic hyphema. Am J Ophthalmol 81:355–360, 1976.
12. McGetrick JJ, Jampol LM, Goldberg MF, Frenkel M, Fiscella RG: Aminocaproic acid decreases secondary hemorrhage after traumatic hyphema. Arch Ophthalmol 101:1031–1033, 1983.
13. Palmer D, Goldberg MF, Frenkel M, Fischella R, Anderson R: Epsilon aminocaproic acid and the prevention and management of secondary traumatic hyphemas: a comparison of two dose regimens. (In press.)
14. Sears ML: Surgical management of black ball hyphema. Trans Am Acad Ophthalmol Otolaryngol 74:820–827, 1970.
15. Edwards WC, Layden WE: Monocular versus binocular patching in traumatic hyphema. Am J Ophthalmol 76:359–362, 1973.
16. Brodrick JD: Corneal blood staining after hyphaema. Br J Ophthalmol 56:589–593, 1972.
17. Wolter JR, Henderson JW, Talley TW: Histopathology of a black ball blood clot removed four days after total traumatic hyphema. J Pediatr Ophthalmol 8:15–17, 1971.

18. Rakusin W: Traumatic hyphema. Am J Ophthalmol 74:284–292, 1972.
19. Lieppman M, Goldberg MF: The treatment of postoperative hyphema by cyclodiathermy. Surv Ophthalmol 26:253–256, 1982.
20. Deutsch TA, Weinreb RN, Goldberg MF: Indications for surgical management of hyphema in patients with sickle cell trait. Arch Ophthalmol 102:566–569, 1984.
21. Goldberg MF: The diagnosis and treatment of sickled erythrocytes in human hyphemas. Trans Am Ophthalmol Soc 76:481–501, 1978.
22. Howard GM, Hutchinson BT, Frederick AR Jr: Hyphema resulting from blunt trauma: gonioscopic, tonographic, and ophthalmoscopic observations following resolution of the hemorrhage. Trans Am Acad Ophthalmol Otolaryngol 69:294–306, 1965.
23. Mooney D: Anterior chamber angle tears after non-perforating injury. Br J Ophthalmol 56:418–424, 1972.
24. Wolff SM, Zimmerman L: Chronic secondary glaucoma: associated with retrodisplacement of iris root and deepening of the anterior chamber and angle secondary to contusion. Am J Ophthalmol 54:547–563, 1962.
25. Milauskas AT, Fueger GF: Serious ocular complications associated with blowout fractures of the orbit. Am J Ophthalmol 62:670–672, 1966.
26. Jensen AD, Cross HE, Paton D: Ocular complications in the Weill-Marchesani syndrome. Am J Ophthalmol 77:261–267, 1974.
27. Chandler PA: Choice of treatment in dislocation of the lens. Arch Ophthalmol 71:765–786, 1964.
28. Jarrett WH II: Dislocation of the lens: a study of 166 hospitalized cases. Arch Ophthalmol 78:289–296, 1967.
29. Barraquer J: Surgery of the dislocated lens. Trans Am Acad Ophthalmol Otolaryngol 76:44–59, 1972.
30. Boniuk M: A new technique for removal of subluxated lenses. Trans Am Acad Ophthalmol Otolaryngol 78:OP60–OP64, 1974.
31. Maumanee AE, Ryan SJ: Aspiration technique in the management of the dislocated lens. Am J Ophthalmol 68:808–811, 1969.
32. Peyman GA, Saunders D: Vitreous and vitreous surgery. In Principles and Practice of Ophthalmology. Peyman GA, Sanders D, Goldberg MF, eds; Philadelphia, WB Saunders Co, 1980, 1364–1390.
33. Cherry PMH: Rupture of the globe. Arch Ophthalmol 88:498–507, 1972.
34. Barr CC: Prognostic factors in corneoscleral lacerations. Arch Ophthalmol 101:919–924, 1983.
35. DeJuan E, Sternberg P, Michaels RG: Penetrating ocular injuries: Types of injuries and visual results. Ophthalmology 90:1318–1322, 1983.
36. Hutton WL, Fuller DG: Factors influencing final visual results in severely injured eyes. Am J Ophthalmol 97:715–722, 1984.
37. Duke-Elder S, MacFaul PA: System of Ophthalmology. Vol. XIV, Injuries. St. Louis, C. V. Mosby Co, 1972.
38. Cox MS, Schepens CL, Freeman HM: Retinal detachment due to ocular compression. Arch Ophthalmol 76:678–685, 1966.
39. Ross WH: Traumatic retinal dialysis. Arch Ophthalmol 99:1371–1377, 1981.
40. Weidenthal DT, Schepens CL: Peripheral fundus changes associated with ocular contusion. Am J Ophthalmol 62:465–477, 1966.
41. Aaberg TM, Blair CJ, Gass JDM: Macular holes. Am J Ophthalmol 69:555–562, 1970.
42. Fuller B, Gitter KA: Traumatic rupture with late serous detachment of macula: report of successful argon laser treatment. Arch Ophthalmol 89:354–355, 1973.
43. Richards RD, West CE, Meisels AA: Chorioretinitis sclopetaria. Am J Ophthalmol 66:852–860, 1968.
44. Duane TD: Valsalva hemorrhagic retinopathy. Am J Ophthalmol 75:637–642, 1973.
45. AtLee WE Jr: Talc and cornstarch emboli in eyes of drug abusers. JAMA 219:49–51, 1972.
46. Kelley JS: Purtscher's retinopathy related to chest compression by safety belts. Am J Ophthalmol 74:278–283, 1972.
47. Marr WG, Marr EG: Some observations on Purtscher's disease: traumatic retinal angiopathy. Am J Ophthalmol 54:693–705, 1962.
48. Ravin JG, Meyer RF: Fluorescein angiographic findings in a case of traumatic asphyxia. Am J Ophthalmol 75:643–647, 1973.

11

Blunt Injuries of the Orbit

When a blunt object strikes the orbit, fractures of the bony orbit may occur. These injuries are discussed in Chapter 3. However, injuries to other structures within the orbit may also occur.

11.1 INJURIES TO THE OPTIC NERVE

Any patient with a history of head trauma, loss of consciousness, or suspected intracranial hemorrhage should have an examination of the optic nerveheads, and the description should be noted in the hospital record. In addition, the pupillary examination is especially important in cases of head injury because the optic nerve can be damaged posterior to the globe and leave no ophthalmoscopically apparent lesion. The presence of a pupillary abnormality may be the only evidence that the visual pathway has been injured. Optic disc pallor is usually not present for two to three weeks.

a. Contusion Injuries

Contusion injuries of the optic nerves are frequently observed.[1-3] The commonest cause of *indirect* injury to the optic nerve is blunt trauma over

215

the anterior skull, especially the brow of the affected eye. Holographic studies of blows to the superolateral area of the brow reveal that the forces tend to be transmitted directly to the optic canal.[3] Such an injury may result in a canalicular fracture with laceration of the optic nerve by a bony fragment as well as compression by a depressed fracture or an intracanalicular hematoma. A variety of visual field losses may occur, but when the defect is altitudinal, the inferior field is more commonly involved, probably as a result of infracture of the superior bony canaliculus.

Traumatic lesions of the chiasm (with bilateral visual field defect as the primary clue) are usually the result of vertex impacts with lines of force directed downward through the chiasm. Direct midline frontal injury may also produce chiasmal trauma of an indirect type.[4]

The secondary effects of indirect trauma to the optic nerves and chiasm result from perineural edema, which may be caused by the contusion itself or by hypoxia from any cause. In this case, the visual field deficit may not be apparent to the patient until hours after the injury, as opposed to the sudden loss associated with laceration or compression as discussed previously.

The treatment of optic nerve injuries is usually expectant. Although claims have been made that high-dose, parenteral corticosteroids are indicated to reduce compressive swelling around the injured nerve,[3] there is no experimental evidence in favor of such treatment. It seems reasonable to administer oral corticosteroids in the usual doses used to reduce cerebral edema. Prednisone in a dose of 60 to 80 mg per day or dexamethasone in a dose of 4 mg every six hours is sufficient.

The question of emergency surgical unroofing of the optic canals after indirect trauma, in hope of preventing edema and necrosis of the optic nerves, has not been resolved. Actual surgical experience with decompression of the canal in some series has only rarely resulted in return of vision.[5] In other series, surgical decompression appears to have been effective.[3, 6] Such surgery carries significant morbidity and mortality and should be undertaken only after carefully weighing the potential benefit to the patient against the risks of blindness or death.

b. Avulsion of the Optic Nerve

Avulsion of the optic nerve results in sudden, permanent, and usually complete loss of vision (see Figure 6–7). There is usually peripapillary hemorrhage and an excavated papilla.[7] Interestingly, the retinal circulation may remain largely intact, whereas the nerve substance is torn completely from the globe. The injury is probably most often caused by a "yo-yo" effect of the globe suddenly moving forward while the optic nerve stays temporarily tethered in place. However, an experimental model for this hypothesis is lacking at the present time.

c. Occult Laceration of the Optic Nerve

When a patient suffers sudden loss of vision and an afferent pupillary defect is present, a careful search should be made for an occult puncture wound around the orbit. A small knife, stiletto, or ice pick can enter the orbit leaving barely a trace and can partially or completely transect the optic nerve. If this occurs posterior to the entrance of the central retinal artery (about 15 mm posterior to the globe), the blood supply will not be injured, and the appearance of the optic disc may be normal.

11.2 INJURIES OF THE EXTRAOCULAR MUSCLES

Motility disturbances following blunt orbital injuries are very common. The examiner is challenged to determine the etiology of the dysfunction.

a. Orbital Hematomas

Hematomas of the extraocular muscles are not uncommon after orbital contusion injuries or lacerations. These hemorrhages are visible only during an exploratory operation, except when the hemorrhage extends along the muscle sheath to the insertion of the tendon on the globe. The only significant consequences of such hemorrhages are the transient limitation of the muscle's action and the problems in differential diagnosis raised thereby. Such problems are usually resolved through the use of the forced-duction test (see Chapter 3).

Diffuse hematomas within the orbit, especially if the muscle cone is involved, may result in a "frozen globe." The eye may appear to be exophthalmic, and the intraocular pressure may be elevated. A conscious patient may complain of profound loss of vision that is often intermittent at first (one form of amaurosis fugax), indicating impending but still reversible early central retinal artery occlusion.

Central retinal artery occlusion causes a characteristic fundus appearance: a pale optic nervehead, narrow arteries (which may show segmentation of their blood columns in severe cases), and diffuse retinal whitening causing a cherry-red spot at the macula where retinal thinness permits transmission of normal choroidal coloration. The cherry-red spot begins to appear within 20 minutes after the occlusion.[8]

Treatment is effective only in those unusual circumstances when a patient is examined within several minutes or hours of the occlusion. Therapy should be started immediately. If the intraocular pressure is elevated, a lateral canthotomy (see below) should be done to relieve the orbital pressure created by the orbital hematoma. Retrobulbar injection of hyaluronidase has been suggested as a means of dissipating orbital edema or blood, but in practice it probably only serves to *increase* the volume of fluid compressing the artery. Paracentesis of the anterior chamber is the most rapid way to decompress the eye and may result in opening a previously closed retinal artery with immediate restoration of arterial pulsations or total perfusion. Intermittent digital massage of the globe is another means of lowering the intraocular pressure (thereby enhancing whatever intravascular head of pressure exists in the central retinal artery).

b. Laceration or Avulsion of Muscles

The ocular muscles are usually not avulsed, but penetrating trauma can sever the muscles or injure their nerve supply or both and thereby render them functionless. The same causes can underlie the limitation of gaze seen in blow-out fractures of the orbit (see Chapter 3). *The presence of focal limitation of gaze should always suggest a penetrating scleral injury*, and this possibility must be ruled out in all cases.

Avulsion of rectus muscles also deprives the anterior segment of its normal blood supply via the anterior ciliary artery accompanying each muscle. If enough of the blood supply is impaired, ischemic necrosis of the anterior segment of the eye can occur. This rarely results from trauma in which the globe itself is preserved, but any reduction of blood supply to an eye with other problems (orbital hemorrhage, carotid-cavernous fistula, sickle cell disease) could be a contributing factor to anterior segment ischemia.

The hemorrhage and swelling accompanying an orbital wound may mask damage to the extraocular muscles, whose action can be greatly limited by orbital swelling alone. Traumatic disinsertion of the muscle tendon may lead to the appearance of tendon fragments in the wound; the muscle belly may be transected or there may be an incomplete tenotomy.

If transection of an extraocular muscle occurs, the muscle frequently contracts toward the orbital apex. Finding the cut end may be difficult, but it is important for proper reconstruction. Injection of a dilute epinephrine solution into Tenon's fascia may induce enough contrast between the red muscle tissue and the blanched subconjunctival connective tissue so that discovery of the muscle is aided. Searching between the bared sclera and Tenon's fascia usually fails to locate the muscle, which has retracted into the loose subconjunctival tissue. Thus, incision of this tissue is usually necessary. Alternatively, simple anterior traction on Tenon's fascia may pull the muscle into view.

In this regard, the problem of adequate surgical exposure at the time of all ocular surgery should be mentioned. A striking difference between experienced and inexperienced surgeons is the relative frequency of poor exposure in the latter's hands. Obviously, inadequate visualization has a significant effect on the success of the operation and often accounts for unnecessary prolongation of the surgery.

Good surgical exposure is particularly vital when seeking an avulsed extraocular muscle or an orbital foreign body; it is also important during surgery posterior to the equator of the eye. *Lateral canthotomy* (performed by first clamping the skin at the lateral canthus and then cutting it with straight scissors) is a first step toward improving exposure of the posterior aspect of the globe. Another helpful maneuver is the use of cotton-tipped applicators to bluntly dissect Tenon's fascia from the rectus muscles as far posteriorly as possible. Finally, the use of traction sutures placed under the rectus muscles and the employment of various retractors generally provide the desired exposure.

Damage to orbital nerves is rare, but stab wounds of the orbit may lead to severance of the optic nerve and isolated paralysis of the oculomotor nerve; a direct injury to the abducens nerve is not uncommon with deep penetrating wounds. However, most traumatic ocular motility impairments (aside from limitations clearly attributable to *orbital* disease) are due to intracranial rather than orbital injuries. In distinction to a positive forced-duction test (see Chapter 3) or even the minimal resistance of normal ocular muscle tonus in a negative test, nerve damage (orbital or intracranial) and severed ocular muscles lead to what might be called a "supranormal" forced duction away from the field of action of the flaccid muscle.

References

1. Walsh FB: Pathological-clinical correlations: I. Indirect trauma to the optic nerves and chiasm; II. Certain cerebral involvements associated with defective blood supply. Invest Ophthalmol 5:433–449, 1966.
2. Walsh FB, Hoyt WF: *Clinical Neuro-Ophthalmology.* (Third Edition). (3 vols). Baltimore, The Williams & Wilkins Co, 1969, 501–502.
3. Anderson RL, Panje WR, Gross CE: Optic nerve blindness following blunt forehead trauma. Ophthalmology 89:445–455, 1982.
4. McCrary JA III: *Pediatric Oculo-Neural Diseases: Case Studies.* Flushing, NY, Medical Examination Publishing Co, 1973.
5. Schmaltz B, Schurmann K: Traumatic damage of the optic nerve: problems of etiology and operative treatment. Klin Monatsbl Augenheilkd 159:33–51, 1971.
6. Fukado Y: Diagnosis and surgical correction of optic canal fracture after head injury. Ophthalmologica (additamentum) 158:307–314, 1969.
7. Park JH, Frenkel M, Dobbie JG, Choromokos E: Evulsion of the optic nerve. Am J Ophthalmol 72:969–971, 1971.
8. Hayreh SS, Weingeist TA: Experimental occlusion of the central artery of the retina. I. Ophthalmoscopic and fluorescein fundus angiographic studies. Br J Ophthalmol 64:896–912, 1980.

12

Anticipation of Certain Injuries

The diagnosis and management of some injuries are greatly facilitated by awareness and anticipation of specific disease entities. In fact, this principle applies to all medical practice. As a simple example, the physician should know that organic foreign bodies retained in the cornea are more likely to produce fungal infection than metallic foreign bodies. Similarly, organic foreign bodies in the orbit must be removed to prevent chronic suppuration, whereas small inaccessible metallic foreign bodies in the orbit are better left alone. The examiner should know that contusion of an eye wearing a contact lens can displace the contact lens into the upper fornix, where it may be retained for a long time if not sought. A traumatic hyphema often causes a child to be obtunded, and this should be borne in mind before initiating a search for a subdural hematoma or other intracranial abnormality. The appearance and behavior of teenagers and young adults with acute loss of vision in one eye may suggest that self-administered intravenous drugs have led to septic retinopathy. In the following pages, certain specific abnormalities will be discussed that require special awareness or suspicion on the part of the physician for either diagnosis or prophylaxis.

12.1 SELF-INFLICTED INJURIES

Whether related to true Oedipism, to masochism, or simply to the need for attention and sympathy, self-inflicted ocular injuries are far more frequent than the uninitiated observer might imagine.[1] The injuries of certain accident-prone individuals repeatedly affect the eyes. Such individuals often are difficult patients and have prolonged recovery periods with a notable incidence of complications. Related to this theme of a psychological predisposition to injury is the peculiar fact that many patients with eye trauma (especially intraocular bullets) have been found to have ominous tattoos such as "born to lose" (Figure 12–1), "born to die," or "born to raise hell."

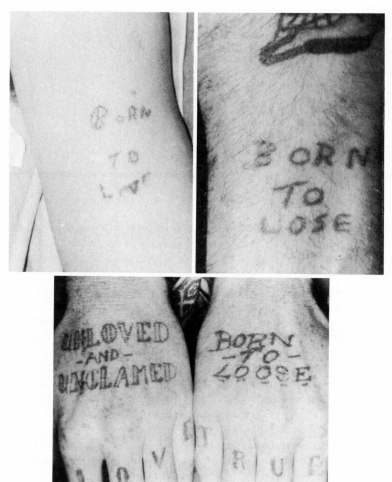

Figure 12–1. There seems to be an interesting relationship between a patient's psychological state and the tendency for recurrent ocular injuries. The tattoos on these three patients sustaining ocular trauma each indicate "born to loose" (lose), and one of these was converted to a new slogan, "born to love."

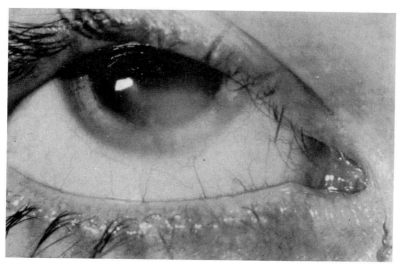

Figure 12–2. Self-inflicted injury to the cornea characterized by epithelial defect and stromal edema. Note that the injury is located on the lower portion of the cornea where the eye is more easily rubbed because of Bell's phenomenon.

a. Corneal Injuries

For whatever reason, some individuals (usually teenagers or young adults) intentionally rub or scratch their eyes with the purpose of causing damage. Since the medical history of such patients is often vague and inconsistent, only a high index of suspicion will lead to diagnosis. Sometimes there will be an admission that a similar "accident" has occurred in the past. Typically, the patient is in pain but is inappropriately unconcerned. Self-inflicted injuries of the cornea should be suspected whenever a lesion seems incompatible with the history, is atypical in nature, and *is located on the lower half of the cornea* (Figure 12–2). While the wound is inflicted, the patient must hold the lids open against a natural tendency to squeeze; this is associated with elevation of the eye (Bell's phenomenon); leaving only the inferior portion of the cornea available for injury.

b. Foreign Substances

Foreign materials of all sorts have been intentionally applied to eyes for a host of reasons.[2] Children wishing to avoid school examinations have used toothpaste as though it were eye ointment, producing punctate staining of the corneal epithelium and conjunctival hyperemia. Dilated and fixed pupils, either unilateral or bilateral, can result from the clandestine use of a cycloplegic medication such as atropine. Foreign substances are usually introduced by pulling down on the lower lid and placing the material in or near the inferior cul-de-sac. Thus, the resultant injury again affects the lower portion of the globe in almost every instance. One extraordinary case of self-inflicted injury was the result of repeated topical administration of pulverized aspirin tablets,[3] leading to the total loss of one eye and impending loss of the second through progressive corneal ulceration (Figure 12–3).

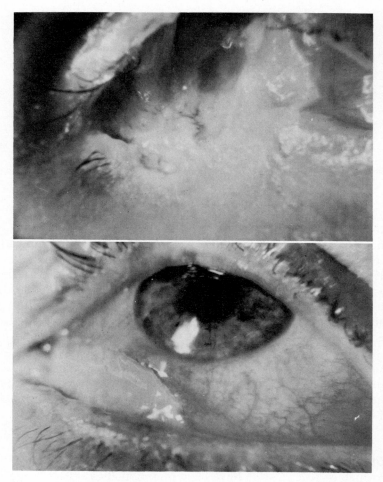

Figure 12–3. The right orbit and left eye of a 34-year-old woman. The patient's right eye was lost after prolonged inflammatory disease of unknown origin, and the left eye shows progressive ulceration extending from the inferior fornix toward the limbus. It was eventually determined that the patient was placing aspirin in the inferior cul-de-sac, causing a gradually progressive mutilation of her only eye—presumably the same procedure as that which led to loss of the right eye. (Case previously reported; photographs reproduced by permission of Copenhaver RM: A report of an unusual self-inflicted eye injury. Arch Ophthalmol, *63*:266–272, 1960.)

c. Autoenucleation

The epitome of classic Oedipism is autoenucleation or autoeviseration of the globe. Such patients are usually transferred from psychiatric institutions with ruptured globes. The presence of blood and intraocular contents beneath the fingernails is a clue to the self-inflicted nature of the injury. Because there is often extensive loss of intraocular contents, the prognosis is generally quite poor. Enucleation of eyes as a punishment rite has also been reported.[4]

d. Sun Gazing

In the presence of acute loss of vision in one or both eyes associated with a tiny white spot or localized edema of the macula, the examiner should suspect solar viewing, either gazing at the sun or observing an eclipse. If the cause is the latter, the lesion is accidental (see Chapter 5), and if it is the former, the lesion is self-inflicted (see Figure 5–7). There are several reports of foveo-macular retinitis occurring in young military personnel, a number of whom wanted to avoid overseas assignments during wartime. Such macular burns from sun gazing may, according to the patient's choice, be unilateral or bilateral. Only the central field of vision is impaired, but this may constitute a profound reduction in acuity, some of which may be permanent. If a patient has an amblyopic eye or lacks fusion, the injured eye is invariably the better eye.

12.2 MALINGERING AND HYSTERIA

Temporarily disturbed, neurotic, or psychotic individuals of all ages may complain of visual loss (minimal or profound) in one or both eyes despite a completely normal examination. No effort will be made here to provide guidelines for the differentiation of malingering from hysteria, for the distinction often is subtle or merely academic. Medicolegal implications incriminate malingering; hysteria is far more likely to occur in high-strung individuals, particularly if there has been some recent physical or psychological trauma to the patient, a close relative, or a close friend.

It is rare that the patient claims no light perception, but the limited acuity being professed invariably is well below the patient's ability to function in our visually oriented world. For instance, a woman may claim hand-motions vision in both eyes yet be able to elegantly apply her own makeup. A man may stumble into the examination room yet aggressively reach out to shake the examiner's hand.

Responses to optokinetic nystagmus testing, normal or excessively abnormal pupillary responses (self-administered atropine), and many tricks by a skilled examiner confirm the diagnosis.[5] A visually evoked potential test, if normal, is very helpful in ruling out organic disease.

Caution must be exercised in interpreting an abnormal test, however, as deliberate inattention on the part of a normal patient can lead to unusual or abnormal wave forms.

Great caution must be taken to rule out retrobulbar neuritis (usually unilateral with an afferent pupillary defect) or occipital cortical blindness (bilateral with normal pupillary reflexes).

12.3 INFLICTED AND IATROGENIC INJURIES

a. Child Abuse

Whereas injuries in the adult eye due to assault are usually identified by the history, the same is not true for infants and small children. For the sake of the future health of the baby, any infant with an eye injury should be suspected of having been abused or neglected. A history of previous injuries or evidence of ecchymoses, fractures, or neglect should reinforce the possibility of this diagnosis and lead to further interviews with parents. If suspicion is high, a report should be made to the legal authorities. In most states, such reporting is mandated by law, and a physician who fails to do so may be subject to criminal charges.

Intentionally traumatized infants often have grossly obvious injuries all over their heads and bodies, some of which may be life-threatening. A search must be made for broken bones, and if the child is obtunded or has focal neurologic signs, a CT scan is indicated to rule out subdural, subarachnoid, or intracranial hemorrhage. The assistance of a pediatrician is invaluable in the diagnosis and treatment of these suspected injuries.

Hyphema, lid lacerations, cataract, dislocated lens, vitreous and retinal hemorrhage, papilledema, and even chemical or thermal burns can be manifestations of adult or sibling hostility. Both parents should be interviewed, not with indignation but with compassion, for one of them may be suffering from a mental illness that must be uncovered for the parent's and the child's sake. If the physician is uncomfortable conducting such an interview, an immediate consult to a social service agency is indicated.

b. Iatrogenic Injuries During Hospital Care

Physicians performing anesthesia or surgery with patients in the face-down position must be constantly aware of the danger of compressing the eye and causing central retinal artery occlusion.[6] Similar compression is also a danger in orbital and lacrimal sac surgical procedures (e.g., blow-out fracture repair[7]). *A patient awakening from such an operative procedure complaining of impaired vision must be managed as a first priority emergency.*

Prevention of ocular compression is, needless to say, far more effective than is the treatment of central retinal artery occlusion. Patients requiring tight bandages after major lid or orbital surgery should have their vision checked every few hours during the first postoperative day, because delayed hematoma formation may induce compression of the optic nerve and central retinal artery. Such hematomas must be decompressed.

When a person is in either the prone or the supine position for general anesthesia, corneal abrasions may easily occur from a variety of ordinarily insignificant factors. If a patient complains of a foreign-body sensation on awakening from anesthesia, a corneal abrasion should be sought and, if detected, treated promptly to avoid development of a corneal ulcer (see Chapter 7). Prior to general surgery, bland ointment is placed over the cornea, and the eyelids should be taped closed. A metal shield may be placed over the eye for protection against inadvertent trauma to the globe.

Rarely, a person with an anatomically narrow anterior chamber angle will develop an attack of acute angle-closure glaucoma as a result of general anesthesia or during the course of hospitalization. Various factors may contribute to the condition: severe anxiety, routine dilatation of the pupils for fundus examination, or preoperative use of systemic atropine. Glaucoma of this nature is readily diagnosed. The pressure is usually markedly elevated (over 30 mm Hg); the cornea may be hazy from edema and the pupil slightly dilated and fixed; the patient generally will complain of aching in the brow, orbit, or eye; decreased vision; and visualization of halos around bright lights. There may also be nausea and vomiting.

Immediate therapy includes pilocarpine-induced miosis, acetazolamide (Diamox) administration, and osmotic therapy (oral glycerin or isosorbide; parenteral mannitol). Once the pressure is restored to normal, the eye (and usually the fellow eye as well) should receive pilocarpine 2% several times a day until a laser or surgical iridotomy can be created.

Surgery on the heart and great vessels or on the head and neck may dislodge emboli that reach the retinal vasculature. Ophthalmic therapy will then involve measures similar to those for central retinal artery occlusion if visual disability occurs.

Paranasal sinus surgery may be complicated unwittingly by optic nerve severance or compression or by damage to the medial wall of the orbit, leading to orbital emphysema with crepitus detected on palpation of the eyelids. Emphysema of the orbit subsides spontaneously.

12.4 OCULAR MANIFESTATIONS OF WHIPLASH INJURY

The pathogenesis and management of whiplash injury and its vague ocular manifestations are poorly understood. Symptomatic of whiplash injury (also called "acute traumatic cervical syndrome") are multiple, nondescript, and sometimes rather persistent complaints that resemble those of mild brain concussion.[8] The precipitating cause is usually a rear-end automobile collision, but there is no history of head trauma or loss of consciousness. Patients complain of headaches, pain and discomfort in the neck, nausea, dizziness, and a variety of ocular discomforts. Blurred vision, eye strain, photophobia, and double vision may accompany a sense of depression and anxiety. While the eye examination is usually normal, anisocoria, precipitous presbyopia, decompensated phorias, vitreous detachment, impaired convergence, ptosis, and ocular fatigue—sometimes transitory and at other times evidently permanent—have all been reported. Each finding and complaint should be managed as if it were unrelated to a symptom complex.

Familiarity with whiplash injury and its ocular manifestations is of great importance in the diagnosis and management of affected individuals. Usually, the patient will point out that litigation is anticipated or in progress. Cognizance of the possibility of malingering, however, should not prejudice the sympathetic care that most of these patients require.

References

1. Brown BZ: Self-inflicted injuries of the eye. Ann Ophthalmol 4:147–158, 1972.
2. Segal P, Mrzyglod S, Alichniewicz-Czaplicka H, Dunin-Horkawicz W, Zwyrzykowski F: Self-inflicted eye injuries. Am J Ophthalmol 55:349–362, 1963.
3. Copenhaver RM: A report of an unusual self-inflicted eye injury. Arch Ophthalmol 63:266–272, 1960.
4. Arago J, cited by Holmes WJ: Avulsion of both eyes: a form of old Hawaiian punishment. Arch Ophthalmol 87:443, 1973.
5. Kramer KK, LaPiana FG, Appleton B: Ocular malingering and hysteria: diagnosis and management. Surv Ophthalmol 24:89–96, 1979.
6. Jampol LM, Goldbaum M, Rosenberg M, Bahr R: Ischemia of posterior ciliary arterial circulation from ocular compression. Arch Ophthalmol 93:1311–1317, 1975.
7. Emery JM, Huff JD, Justice J Jr: Central retinal artery occlusion after blow-out fracture repair. Am J Ophthalmol 78:538–540, 1974.
8. Roca PD: Ocular manifestations of whiplash injuries. Ann Ophthalmol 4:63–73, 1972.

Index

Note: Page numbers in *italics* refer to illustrations; page numbers followed by (t) refer to tables.